Dash Diet Cookbook

Quick and Easy Recipes to Rapidly Reduce Hypertension

Alvin Ray

Table of contents

Introduction

Hypertension remains the most important cause of death worldwide. But via therapy and dietary change, it is preventable. Hypertension management methods consist of dietary modifications including a diet high in fruits, low-fat foods or fish and vegetables with a reduced saturated and total fat content, limited salt intake, regular exercise, appropriate body weight, less alcohol consumption, and drug therapies, even though these differ to some extent according to various published treatment guidelines for hypertension.

Starting the DASH diet is one of the moves your doctor might prescribe to reduce your high blood pressure.

DASH is abbreviated as "Dietary approaches to stop hypertension". The DASH diet is intended to treat or avoid elevated blood pressure (hypertension) and is a comprehensive strategy to have healthy nutrition. In studies funded by the National Institutes of Health, the DASH diet strategy was designed to reduce blood pressure without medicine. Vegetables and low-fat dairy foods are favored in the DASH diet, as well as the optimum number of whole grains, poultry, nuts and fishes.

There is also a reduced salt variant of the diet, in addition to the regular DASH diet. You should pick the diet variant that suits your requirements for health.

The DASH diet helps you lower the sodium concentration in the daily routine diet and enables you to enjoy several nutrient-rich foods that contain potassium, magnesium and calcium to lower the blood pressure.

You could be able to reduce the blood pressure by a few steps in approximately two weeks by adopting the DASH diet. Your high blood pressure (the systolic) can decrease by 8 - 14 points with the time that can make a considerable difference to your health risks.

Since the DASH diet is a safe way of eating, it not only reduces blood pressure but also provides cardiovascular benefits.

For the treatment of cancer, osteoporosis, heart disease, diabetes and stroke, the DASH diet is also in suggestion with nutritional guidelines.

Chapter 1 – DASH Diet

1.1 Origin

Dietary Methods to avoid Hypertension (DASH) emerged in the 1990s. The National Institute of Health (NIH) began funding a variety of research studies in 1992 to see that particular dietary approaches are effective in the treatment of hypertension or not. To prevent any potential factors, the study participants were recommended to follow only the dietary treatments and not include any other lifestyle changes. They observed that systolic blood pressure could only be lowered by around 6 to 11 mmHg by dietary activity alone. This influence was shown in persons with both hypertension and normotension. In several cases, the DASH diet centered upon these findings has been advised as the first-line therapy with a lifestyle change.

1.2 What is used in this diet?

DASH encourages the intake of fruits, vegetables, lean meat and milk items and the use of micro-nutrients in the menu. The lowering of sodium in the diet to around 1500 mg/day is often advo-cated. DASH focuses on the consumption of food that is minimally refined and fresh. There are also similarities between the DASH diet and some of the other nutritional strategies advocated for cardiovascular fitness. The DASH diet is an apogee of the modern world, as well as ancient times. Scientists have mined it on the basis of some ancient culinary principles, and it has been adapted to target some of the leading causes of mortality and morbidity in the modern world.

1.3 Enhancing Healthcare Team Outcomes

For controlling hypertension, the DASH diet is a nutritionally balanced approach. In many clinical trials, the diet has been studied and found to reduce saturated fats, blood pressure and cholesterol. DASH diet has been prescribed as the safest diet for those who wish to lose weight and reduce blood pressure. The real criterion is that the patients must be encouraged to this diet. Both nurses and pharmacists play a vital role in teaching the patients about the effects of this diet in addition to doctors. Nurses are in a perfect role. They can teach both patients and family members more about the DASH diet and its advantages right before discharge.

Similarly, the pharmacist should teach the customer about the DASH diet while patients visit a pharmacy. The DASH diet's most critical features are that it needs a lifestyle transition and a healthier way to eat. In conjunction, patients should be advised to avoid smoking, refrain from alcohol, and actively engage in any physical exercise.

1.4 Is the DASH diet primarily preferred for Hypertension care only?

It has been researched thoroughly to check the DASH diet's treatment paradigm and its effects on several other diseases.

Several studies have found that the DASH diet improves by reducing triglycerides, LDL-C, blood glucose levels, as well as insulin tolerance. Such behavior allows the DASH diet to significantly contribute to metabolic syndrome's pharmacological treatment (a major epidemic in this region). It has also become a powerful element for weight control. Complying some populations with the DASH diet has demonstrated substantial changes in type 2 diabetes treatment. Its focus on lowering dietary sodium and promoting the consumption of calcium, potassium, and magnesium, which is a recommended diet in patients with heart disease.

1.5 Research and general acceptance

Reports have indicated that excessive salt consumption plays a role in high blood pressure progression over the years. Dietary recommendations for the avoidance and control of hypertension have mostly centered on reducing sodium or salt consumption. In 1989, a study scrutinized the reaction of 3 to12 g of salt consumption per day to blood pressure. This study showed that a small decrease in salt, i.e., 5-6 g of salt a day, allows the blood pressure to decrease in patients with hypertension. The better result was shown with just 3 g of salt a day intake, with a mean drop in blood pressure of systolic (11 mmHg) and diastolic (6 mmHg), respectively. More notably, the low-salt diets used for high blood pressure reduction or recovery have been questioned. The Phase II Hypertension Prevention Trials in 1997 suggested that energy consumption and weight loss in the prevention of hypertension were more significant than limiting dietary salt. A 2006 Cochrane study (which investigated the effect of a longer-term moderate reduction in salt on blood pressure) observed that a modest decrease in salt consumption could substantially influence blood pressure in individuals with hypertension but a smaller impact on those without blood pressure. It was decided that the 2007 public health guidelines would have a positive impact on blood pressure and cardiovascular disease by reducing salt consumption from 9-12 g / day to a modest level i.e., 5-6 g /day.

The potency of a DASH diet is well known for controlling blood pressure. As an example of a healthy eating schedule (compatible with the 2015 Dietary Guidelines' current recommendations for Americans), proposed the DASH Eating Plan, which constitutes the foundation for USDA MyPlate and their recommendations, such as those promoted by a British Nutrition Foundation, American Society for Hypertension and the American Heart Association also prescribe the DASH.

While lowering sodium and increasing the consumption of potassium, calcium, and magnesium play a crucial role in decreasing blood pressure, but the reasons for the beneficial effects of the DASH eating plan remain unclear. The researchers say that it may be that whole food ingests potassium, calcium, and magnesium, or it may be due to the combined effect of consuming those nutrients collectively rather than the specific nutrients individually. It is also suspected that the link between diet and blood pressure could be another anonymous factor present in fruits, vegetables, and low-fat dairy products.

The Salt Institute encourages the DASH diet but without limiting the salt. They assert that a DASH diet alone would produce the necessary decrease in blood pressure without the decreased sodium consumption from packaged foods. Their suggestion is focused on the reality that no evidence-based findings justify a need for the whole population to limit dietary salt. The 2006 Cochrane review found that a small decrease in salt consumption dramatically reduce blood pressure in hypertension's patient but had little impact on average blood pressure. The salt limitation is not advised for people without hypertension.

1.6 Precautions

To prevent side effects such as gas, bloating, and diarrhea, the addition of high-fiber foods to the diet should be achieved progressively. Increasing fluid at the same time is necessary since fiber pulls water into the intestine. High fibers consumption can induce hard stools and constipation with insufficient fluid.

The rise in fruits and vegetables improves the diet's potassium content. A higher intake of potassium from foods presents little risk for healthy people with proper kidney function because extra potassium is excreted in the urine. However, there may be a chance of hyperkalemia (high potassium levels in the blood) in people whose urinary potassium excretion is compromised, such as patients with end-stage renal disease, significant cardiac failure or adrenal insufficiency. Hyperkalemia can lead to an erratic heartbeat (cardiac arrhythmia), which can be dangerous. Also, some popular medications may minimize the excretion of potassium. Before beginning the DASH diet, patients at risk should contact a doctor since a higher intake of potassium in the form of fruit and vegetables might not be sufficient. For the substitution of potassium-containing salt, caution should also be taken.

1.7 Risks

There are no known complications linked with the DASH diet currently. The long-term impacts of the diet on illness and mortality are still uncertain.

Chapter 2 – Sample menus for the DASH diet

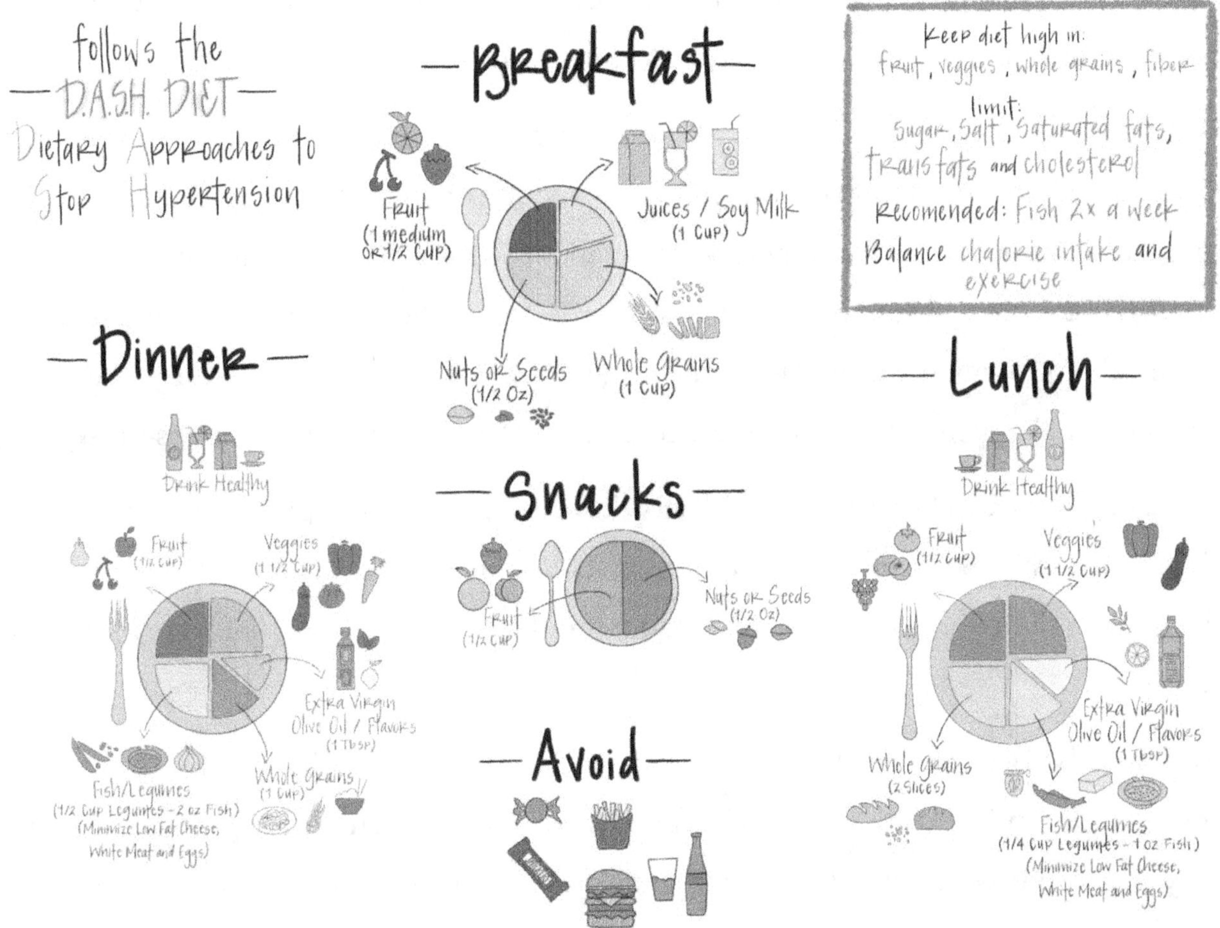

2.1 Involved in implementing the eating schedule for DASH, but how?

The DASH diet includes menus containing whole foods, seafood, meat and nuts, lots of greens, fruits and low-fat dairy products. Small portions of red meat, desserts and drinks are also offered.

You may like to try the DASH diet, but you're not sure how to combine DASH into your regular menus. Here are the menus, conforming to the DASH schedule to help you get started. As a basis for your balanced meal plans, use these menus.

Remember that you may eat a few more or a few smaller portions on certain days than prescribed for a specific food category. That's normally fine, as far as the guidelines are similar to the average of a few days or even a week. The exception is that of sodium. Aim to remain as close to the daily sodium level as possible. Notice also that nutritional content values can differ based on the particular brands of ingredients you use or alterations you make in preparing meals.

Formulating the DASH diet aims to reduce blood pressure and to diminish the risk of heart disease. In developed nations, heart disease remains the leading cause of death in males and females, and meaningful actions can be taken to significantly decrease its chances.

That's because all of the heart disease risk factors are largely within our control. They include actively participating in inappropriate exercise, preventing obesity and eating a balanced diet. For starters, merely removing added sugars from the diet will reduce the risk. It can also greatly impact your risk profile by eating more fruits, vegetables and whole grains and eating less refined and red meat. Too many sugars and too much meat intake is associated with reduced health. Conversely, it would be helpful to replace these ingredients with more nutritious substitutes.

Persons using the DASH diet in clinical trials decreased their blood pressure after two weeks. Another diet, DASH-Sodium, allows sodium to be downsized to 1,500 mg per day (approximately 2/3 of a teaspoon). Studies of individuals on the DASH-Sodium diet have reduced their blood pressure.

Starting the DASH Diet: The DASH diet needs a few numbers of daily servings from different food groups. Depending on the number of calories you require each day, the number of servings can vary that you need. It would be best if you made incremental alterations. For example: start by restricting yourself to 2400 mg of sodium a day (about one teaspoon). Then, cut down to 1500 mg of sodium a day (about 2/3 teaspoons) until the body transitions to the diet. These levels include all absorbed sodium, including sodium consumed in food items and fried things or added to the table.

2.2 Dash Diet Tips

- Add servings of vegetables in lunch and dinner.

- For your dinners or as a snack, add servings of fruit.

- It is quick to use canned and dried fruits, but ensure that they have no added sugar.

- Using just half the traditional butter, salad dressing, margarine serving, and low or fat-free seasonings.

- Drink low-fat or skim dairy items whenever you use cream or full-fat.

- Limit meat to 6 ounces a day. Make some vegetable meals.

- Drink low-fat or skim dairy items where full-fat or cream is usually used.

- Restrict the amount of meat to 6 ounces daily.

- Have some veggie meals.

- Add more dried beans and fruits to your daily diet.

- Eat unsalted pretzels or almonds, raisins, reduced sugar and fat-free milk, unsalted, plain popcorn without butter, fresh veggies and frozen yogurt instead of snacking sweets and chips.

- To select items that are lower in sodium, read the food labels.

2.4 To continue the DASH Diet

The DASH diet recommends to get:

Grains: 7 to 8 daily servings

Vegetables: 4 to 5 daily servings

Fruits: 4 to 5 daily servings

Low or fat-free milk products: 2 to 3 daily servings

Meat, fish and poultry: 2 or <2 servings

Seeds, nuts and dry beans: 4 to 5 servings a week

Oils and Fats: 2 to 3 daily servings

Sweets: tend to limit < 5 servings a week

Below is a closer look at those guidelines.

Carbohydrates:

Carbohydrates are mostly made up of cellulose and starches in the diet. The human body cannot digest cellulose. It is predominantly found in fiber from plants. In the diet, "carbs" or healthy starches must be included, not just for the availability of calories but also for the defensive micronutrients. Low carb diets are not as safe as this will result in lowered calorie consumption as prescribed or an additional intake of unhealthy fats.

Under DASH, balanced carbohydrates include:

- **Green leafy vegetables: kale, broccoli, spinach, collards and mustards**

- **Legumes and beans**

- **Low glucose index fruits**

- **Whole grains: millets, cracked wheat and oats**

Fats:

Fats are a prime suspect in the advancement of the chronic disease epidemic most of the time. However, research has now proven true. Fats are now classified as good and bad fats.

Good fats supply essential fatty acids, promote overall health and avoid inflammation. These fats have increased HDL and decreased small, dense LDL particles when consumed in moderation. Some of the sources of good fats also included in DASH include:

- **Avocados**

- **Fish rich in omega-3 fatty acids**

- **Flax seeds**

- **Hempseeds**

- **Nuts**

- **Olive oil**

Bad fats, including vegetable shortenings, margarine, partly hydrogenated vegetable oils, induce an increase in atherogenesis-promoting minor LDL particles.

Fats are a heavily concentrated energy supply that has to be eaten in moderation. Thus their serving amounts in the DASH guidelines are much lower than those for other nutrients.

Proteins:

More servings of plant proteins, including soy products, legumes, seeds and nuts, are advised by DASH. In the diet, animal protein can primarily consist of lean meats, eggs, low-fat milk products, and fish. Since they have been shown to induce hypertension and even contain carcinogens, therefore, cured and dried meats are not suggested.

The DASH diet also addresses the use of some foods high in potassium, magnesium and calcium, as they inhibit endothelial dysfunction and facilitate endothelial relaxing of the smooth muscle. Bananas, Spinach and oranges are some of the potassium-rich foods. Calcium is rich in green leafy vegetables and dairy products. In several leafy greens, whole grains, beans and nuts, magnesium is present.

2.3 Change gradually

Add a serving at lunch and another at dinner if you are eating one or two vegetables a day. Add a serving to your meals or have it as a snack, if you do not eat fruit or have only juice at breakfast. Improve your use of fat-free and low-fat milk and milk products gradually to 3 servings a day. Drink milk at lunch or at dinner instead of sugar-sweetened tea, soda or alcohol. To reduce your consumption of saturated fat, the total fat, cholesterol, and calories and boost your calcium, choose fat-free (skimmed) or low fat (1 %) milk products. To choose the lowest saturated fat and trans-fat, read the nutrition facts on salad dressings and margarine.

2.5 Making the DASH to Good Health

A new way of eating for a lifetime is the DASH plan. Don't let it away from accessing your fitness goals if you slip out of the diet pattern for a few days. Return to the track.

Here's how:

Ask yourself why you have been off-track. Has it been at a party? Were you at home or work and feeling stressed? Find out how you divagated and start with the DASH plan again. Yes, don't worry about slipping. Especially when learning something new, everybody slips. Remember that it is a long-term process to change your lifestyle. See if you've tried to do too much all at once. Those who are beginning a new lifestyle often try to change too much at once. Change one or two things at a time instead. It is the best way to succeed, slowly but surely. Break down the cycle into small steps. By doing so, you will not only be stopped to execute excessively at once, but it also makes the modifications simpler. Break complicated objectives into smaller and simpler steps, and each of which is achievable. Write down that. To keep a record of your eaten food and what you're doing. This activity can assist you in finding the issue. Keep track of multiple days. For example, you may find that while watching television, you eat high-fat foods. If so, instead of high-fat foods, you could start keeping a substituted snack on hand to eat. This record also helps you be sure that you get enough of every food group and physical activity every day. Celebrate performance. For your achievements, treat yourselves to a non-food treat.

Chapter 3 – Breakfast Recipes

New literature indicates that eating a too much breakfast, a more moderate lunch, and consuming less meal at dinner time is an eating plan associated with improved weight loss and management for individuals trying to lose (or control) body weight. When we eat most of our daily calories early in the day, it appears we fare better.

In the face of the experiences and traditions of other Americans, this travels. On the run, we prefer to eat breakfast and leave the big meal for the day's end. A safer approach is there. Why not try and eat the most of your calories and allow yourself to enjoy your feast in the morning?

To help you live a healthy life, the DASH Diet focuses on ingredients consumption in the morning to reduce your blood pressure. A significant tip is here: Never, ever, miss breakfast. It is counter-productive, and later in the day, it sets you up for overeating. By choosing a nutritional breakfast to eat, launch your day right off. In this diet plan, healthy breakfast selections include protein, fruits, vegetables, low-fat dairy products and whole grains. Give a lift to your mornings with these delectable recipes.

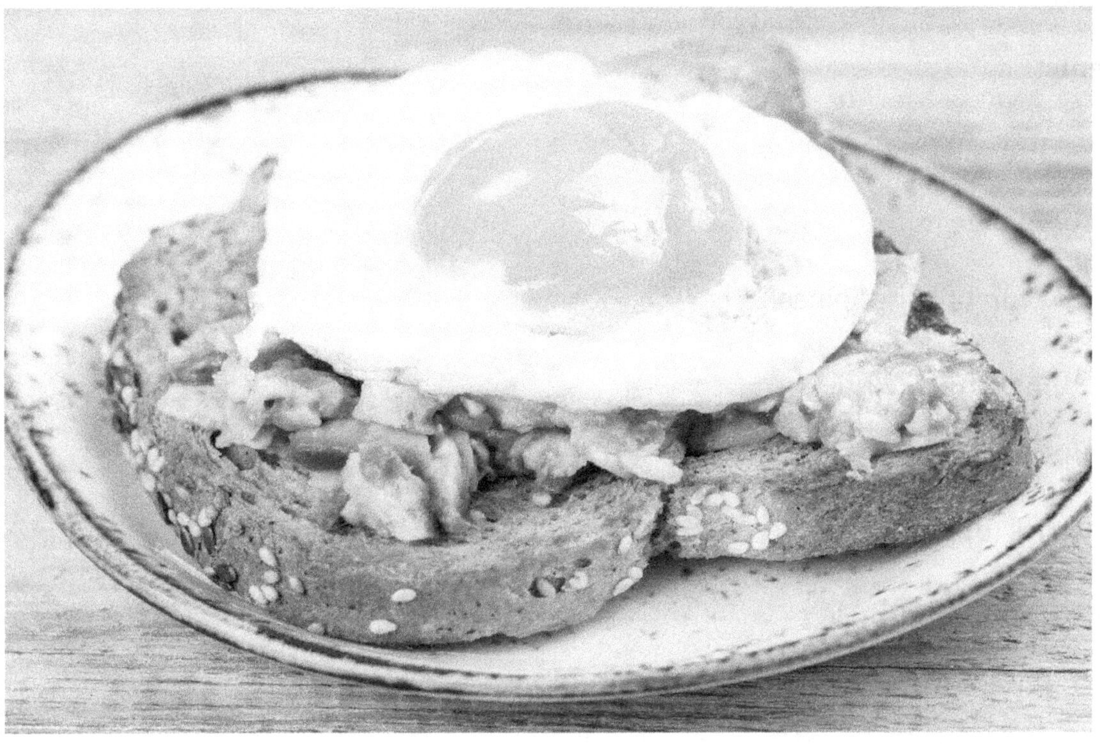

3.1 Almond Butter Berry Smoothie

YIELD: 2 servings

Ingredients

- 1 tablespoon almond butter (creamy)

- 1 cup fresh/frozen raspberries

- 1/2 medium banana (ripe)

- 1/2 cup ice (crushed)

- 1/4 cup low-fat milk (1%)

Directions

Blend until smooth, and then enjoy all the ingredients.

3.2 Spinach Sunshine Smoothie Bowl

YIELD: 1 serving

Ingredients

- 1 banana

- 1 cup of orange juice

- 1 packed cup of baby spinach

- 1/2 avocado

- 1/2 cup of ice cubes

- blueberries (optional)

- diced pineapple (optional)

- ground flaxseeds (optional)

Directions

1. Cook the spinach, avocado, pineapple, orange juice, and ice until it becomes creamy.

2. Filled with sliced ground flaxseeds, pineapple and blueberries and serve.

3.3 Peaches And Pomegranate Avocado Toast

YIELD: 1 serving

Ingredients

- 1 slice of whole-grain bread

- 1 teaspoon ricotta

- pomegranate seeds(small handful)

- honey drizzles

- 1/2 avocado

Directions

1. In the microwave oven or toaster, toast the whole grain bread.

2. Spread avocado (coarse or smooth as you want) on the toast.

3. Spread all over the avocado with a dollop of ricotta.

4. Drizzle over the avocado mixture with a touch of butter.

5. Sprinkle on top of pomegranate seeds and enjoy.

3.4 Breakfast in a Jar

YIELD: 1 serving

Ingredients

- 1 tablespoon of chia seeds

- 2 tablespoon raisins

- 1 tablespoon unsweetened coconut flakes

- 1/4 cup of oatmeal

- 3/4 cup of kefir

Directions:

1. In a 16-ounce mason jar, cover the ingredients, cover the lid, and keep in refrigerate overnight.

2. Take the container from the fridge when it's time to eat and give it a fast stir.

3.5 Avocado Egg Cups

YIELD: 4 servings

Ingredients

- 2 avocados (ripened)

- 4 medium eggs

- 1 tablespoon of grated cheese (like Parmesan, Swiss or cheddar)

- 1/2 tablespoon of olive oil

- 1/4 tablespoon of coarse salt

- 1/4 tablespoon of pepper

Assorted toppings: scallions, herbs, salsa, diced tomato, Sriracha, paprika, crumbled bacon and crumbled feta

Directions:

1. Heat the oven to 375 °F. Halve the avocados and pit lengthwise. Cut a quite thin slice from the bottom of each half of the avocado such that the level lies. Scoop out enough of the flesh (around 1/2 tbsp) and pit it, inorder to make space for an egg.

2. Place the avocados on a rimmed baking sheet lined with foil. Season with pepper and salt, and apply the olive oil to the mixture.

3. Through each cavity, smash an egg (some of the white egg will run over the side, so don't think about it). Sprinkle (if used) with cheese. Cover with foil loosely.

4. Bake for 20 to 25 minutes or until you have your eggs prepared to your taste. And sprinkle with toppings.

3.6 Daphne Oz's Sugar Break Apple and Peanut Butter Oatmeal

YIELD: 4 servings

Ingredients

- 1 cup of steel-cut oats

- peanut butter's swirl

- pinch ground cinnamon

- 1 tablespoon butter (optional)

- 4 cups of water

- Pinch of salt

- 3 medium of large Granny Smith apples (cored and sliced into 1 or 2-inch chunks)

Directions:

1. Process the oats until they hit the thickness and creaminess at the desired level.

2. Chop the apples and toss them with the oats, and then stir.

3. Attach the peanut butter and stir until it is melted and spread all over.

4. Cover the cinnamon and butter with a splash (not mandatory) and enjoy it.

3.7 Sweet Potato Toast

YIELD: 1 serving

Ingredients

- 1 potato (sweet)

Directions

1. Cut into 1/4-inch slices of the sweet potato and put it in the toaster.

2. Top that with anything you want. Nut butter with strawberries, avocado, hummus, eggs, cheese, and tuna salad are common combos.

Note: The amount of calories is based on one sweet potato but does not consider the toppings.

Various toppings will add 25-383 extra calories everywhere. Cut the sweet potato into 1/4-inch slices and pop into the toaster.

3.8 Tofu Turmeric Scramble

YIELD: 2 servings

Ingredients

- ¼ cup of nutritional yeast

- ¼ red onion (chopped)

- ½ cup button mushrooms (sliced)

- ½ tablespoon turmeric

- ½ tablespoon of salt and pepper

- 1 8-ounce block of firm/extra-firm tofu (drained)

- 1 green or red bell pepper (chopped)

- olive oil (extra virgin)

- garlic powder

- 2 cups fresh Spinach (loosely chopped)

Directions

1. To eliminate excess water, clear the tofu and pinch gently. Crumble the tofu by hand into a bowl- the finer pieces will be better.

2. Put a large skillet on medium heat and cook the vegetables. Include the olive oil, onions, and bell peppers when ready. Mix a pinch of the pepper and salt and simmer to soften the vegetables for around 5 minutes. Add the mushrooms and stir-fry for 2 minutes. Add tofu then. Stir-fry for 3 minutes or slightly longer if the tofu is thin.

3. Then add the remaining salt & pepper, garlic, nutritional yeast and turmeric and mix well with a spatula to ensure that spices are well balanced. Cook until the tofu is finely browned, for another 5 to 8 minutes.

4. Add the Spinach and steam for 2 minutes to coat the pan. Serve instantly.

3.9 Ulli's Granelli

YIELD: 26 servings

Ingredients

- 1/2 cup of maple syrup

- 1/3 cup orange oil (pure)

- 1/4 cup coconut oil (unrefined), along with 2 tablespoon for oiling the baking sheet

- 2 cups dried cherries/cranberries

- 2 cups raisins (organic)

- 2 cups almonds (raw)

- 2 cups cashews (raw)

- 2 cups pumpkin seeds (raw)

- 2 cups sunflower seeds (raw)

- 2 cups walnuts (raw)

- 3 cups unsweetened coconut flakes

- 4 cups rolled oats

- pinch of sea salt

Directions

1. Preheat the Microwave oven to 300 degrees Fahrenheit.

2. Combine the peas, almonds, seeds and coconut flakes in a large bowl and blend well.

3. Whisk the maple syrup, salt and coconut oil and orange oil together in a smaller bowl until thoroughly mixed, then spill over the oat-nut mixture and meld well.

4. Spread granola on a large oiled baking sheet (do it in batches if necessary) and bake until golden brown for 35-40 minutes (rotate the baking sheet for even baking halfway through).

5. Remove from the oven and allow to cool fully before melding with cranberries or dried and raisins

6. To preserve additional crispiness, store in airtight containers in the fridge.

3.10 Whole Grain Cottage Cheese Pancakes

YIELD: 4 servings

Ingredients

- 1 cup oat flour

- 2 tbsp teff flour

- 1 tbsp baking powder

- 3 eggs

- 4 tsp canola oil

- 1-pint blueberries

- 1/2 cup sorghum flour

- 1/2 tsp salt

- 3 1/2 tsp sugar

- 1/2 tsp flax meal

- 1/2 tsp vanilla extract

- 1/2 cup maple syrup

- 1/3 cup plus 1 tbsp tapioca starch

- 1/3 cup cottage cheese

- 3/4 cup buttermilk

- 1 tsp lemon juice

- 3 tbsp water

- pinch of salt

Directions:

1. In a wide mixing bowl, combine all of your dried ingredients and stir to combine evenly.

2. In a separate container, mix all of your wet ingredients.

3. Create a well in the center of your dry ingredients and start pouring in the wet ingredients slowly, around a quarter cup at a time. This act will ensure that while whisking, no lumps form.

4. When a smooth batter appears, start to add the wet ingredients to the flour foundation. When you preheat your grill pan, let the butter for 15 minutes at rest.

5. Make a warm maple blueberry compote when the grill heats up. In a small pot, combine the blueberries, maple syrup, water, lemon juice, and salt pinch. For blending, whisk uniformly.

6. Heat the pot gently on low heat till the blueberries begin to pop, and their natural juices are released. Put back, keep it warm.

7. Lightly oil the grill pan using the nonstick spray or use a limited volume of neutral-flavored oil until the grill pan is preheated to a medium-high temperature.

8. Scoop the batter on to the grill pan, and make sure that the griddle is not overcrowded.

9. Enable the pancakes to bake repeatedly until the sides look dry without cracking, and bubbles come to the top. This act should take about two minutes.

10. Turn the pancakes over and cook for another two minutes on the other side.

11. Keep warm or serve with the warm maple-blueberry compote immediately.

3.11 Very Berry Muesli

YIELD: 4 Servings

Ingredients

- Salt (Pinch)

- 1/4 cup toasted walnuts (chopped)

- 1/2 cup blueberries (frozen)

- 1/2 cup of dried fruit such as try raisins, dates and apricots

- 1/2 cup apple (chopped)

- 1/2 cup milk (1%)

- 1 cup of raw old-fashioned rolled oats

- 1 cup of fruit yogurt

Directions

1. Mix the oatmeal, milk, yogurt and salt in a medium dish.

2. For 6-12 hours, cover and refrigerate.

3. Gently mix and add dried and fresh berries.

4. In little bowls, serve spoonful of muesli. Sprinkle with chopped nuts for each meal.

5. Leftovers can be refrigerated within 2-3 hours.

3.12 Red Pepper, Kale, and Cheddar Frittata

YIELD: 6-8 SERVINGS

Ingredients

- 5 oz spinach and baby kale

- 3/4 cup of Milk

- 12 eggs

- 1/4 tablespoon salt

- 1/4 tablespoon pepper

- 1/3 cup sliced scallions

- 1 tablespoon olive oil

- 1 red pepper (diced)

- 1 cup cheddar cheese (sharp shredded)

Directions

1. Preheat the oven to 375 degrees Fahrenheit.

2. Spray with olive oil or nonstick spray on an 8 1/2-inch or 12-inch glass or casserole dish.

3. In a large frying pan, heat the oil. Stir in the red peppers and simmer until tender. Apply the kale and Spinach, stirring regularly or around 3 minutes before the greens are wilted.

4. Move the peppers and greens, scattered thinly to the bowl. Add the sliced scallions.

5. Consolidate the salt, milk, and pepper with the eggs. Over the pan, add the egg mixture. Sprinkle the end of the cheese.

6. Bake for 35-40 minutes, or when the mixture is perfectly set and lightly browned. Place under the broiler for just an additional 1 to 3 minutes to add the color and check thoroughly to ensure that the top does not burn. Until cutting, let it cool for about 5 minutes.

7. Serve it warm, or refrigerate throughout the week for a simple breakfast. Reheat the microwave for 1-2 minutes.

3.13 Veggie Quiche Muffins

YIELD: 12 Servings

Ingredients

- 4 eggs

- 3/4 cup of shredded cheddar cheese (low-fat)

- 2 cups milk (nonfat or 1%)

- 1/2 teaspoon salt

- 1/2 teaspoon pepper

- 1 teaspoon of Italian seasoning (or dried leaf basil & oregano)

- 1 cup tomatoes (diced)

- 1 cup green onion or onion (chopped)

- 1 cup broccoli (chopped)

- 1 cup baking mix (intended for pancakes or biscuits)

Directions:

1. Heat the oven to 375 °F. Lightly spray the12 muffin cups or oil them.

2. Sprinkle the muffin cups with cheese, broccoli, onions and tomatoes.

3. In a pan, put the rest of the ingredients and beat until smooth. In muffin cups, spill the egg mixture over the other ingredients.

4. Bake for 35-40 minutes, until the golden brown or the knife inserted in the middle comes out clean. Cool for five minutes.

5. Leftovers should be refrigerated within 2 hours.

3.14 Sweet Millet Congee

YIELD: 8 Servings

Ingredients

- ¼ cup honey

- 1 cup of hulled millet

- 1 cup peeled and diced sweet potato

- 1 medium diced with skin apple

- 1 teaspoon of ground cinnamon

- 2 tablespoons of brown sugar

- 2 teaspoons of minced ginger (optional)

- 5 cups of water

- 8 bacon's strips

Directions:

1. Cook the bacon in a skillet until it becomes crispy, at medium-high heat. To eliminate extra fat, remove it from the pan and blot it with a paper towel. Crumble the bacon strips until it becomes

cooled, and set aside.

2. Rinse the millet and drain it.

3. In a deep bath, mix the millet, water, ginger, cinnamon, sweet potato, and brown sugar. Ring to a simmering, reduce heat to low and boil until water evaporates (approximately 1 hour) and stirring regularly.

4. If the millet has been baked, remove the pot from the heat and add crumbles of apple, honey and bacon.

5. Method of slow cooking: Lessen the 1 cup water and cook 2 to 21/2 hours on high.

3.15 Turkey Sausage and Mushroom Strata

YIELD: 12 Servings

Ingredients

- ½ cup green onion (chopped)

- ½ teaspoon of paprika

- 1 cup mushrooms (sliced)

- 1-1/2 cup of 4 ounces cheddar cheese (reduced-fat shredded sharp)

- 12 ounces of egg's substitute

- 12 ounces of turkey sausage (can be frozen section)

- 2 cups milk (fat-free)

- 2 tablespoons parmesan cheese (grated)

- 3 large eggs

- 8 ounces of wheat ciabatta bread (1" cubes)

- Fresh ground pepper for taste

Directions

1. Preheat the oven to 400 degrees Fahrenheit.

2. On a baking sheet, place cubes of bread. Bake for 8 minutes at 400 °F or until it becomes toasted.

3. Over the medium-high flame, heat a medium skillet. Add the sausage to the pan; cook for just 7 minutes and stirring to crumble or until browned.

4. Add the milk, eggs, egg substitute, cheese, parmesan cheese, salt, paprika, and pepper with a whisk in a big cup.

5. Add the sausage bread, mushrooms and scallions, and toss to cover the bread well. Do spoon mixing in a 13*9-inch baking pan. Cover it and refrigerate for 8 hours or overnight.

6. Preheat the furnace to 27 °F.

7. Uncover the casserole. Bake for 50 minutes at 350 °F or until lightly browned. Split into 12 pieces and serve instantly.

3.16 Summer Breakfast Quinoa Bowls

YIELD: 2 Servings

Ingredients

- ¾ + 2/3 cup milk (low-fat)

- 2 teaspoons of honey

- 2 teaspoons of brown sugar

- 14 blueberries

- 12 raspberries

- 1/3 cup well-rinsed uncooked quinoa

- 1/2 teaspoon of vanilla extract

- 1 small sliced peach

Directions:

1. In a saucepan, combine quinoa and 2/3 cup milk, vanilla and brown sugar.

2. Cook on medium heat and bring to boil for five minutes. Reduce heat to low and cover it. Cook for 15 to 20 minutes, or until easily fluffs with a fork.

3. Meanwhile, heat a grill pan and spray with oil. Grill the peaches to bring out their sweetness 2 to 3 minutes and set aside. Warm the remaining milk in the microwave.

4. Divide the cooked quinoa between 2 bowls, then pour in warmed milk. Top with peaches, raspberries and blueberries and drizzle each with 1 teaspoon of honey.

3.17 Strawberry Breakfast Sandwich (Halves)

YIELD: 8 Servings

Ingredients

- 1 tablespoon of honey
- 1 teaspoon of grated Lemon zest
- 2 cups 10-ounces strawberries (sliced)
- 4 split and toasted English muffins
- 8-ounces Neufchatel cheese/low-fat softened cream cheese

Directions:

1. In a food processor, process the honey, cheese and zest until they become fully mixed. You can mix in a bowl with a wooden spoon.

2. Unfurl the 1 tablespoon of cheese mixture on the cut side of 1 muffin half and top with 1 quarter cup of strawberries.

3. Perform the same procedure with the remaining ingredients to make eight half-sandwiches.

3.18 Spinach, Mushroom, and Feta Cheese Scramble

YIELD: 1 Serving

Ingredients

- ½ cup fresh sliced mushrooms
- 1 cup fresh chopped Spinach
- 2 egg whites & 1 whole egg

- 2 tablespoons of feta cheese

- Cooking spray

- Pepper for taste

Directions:

1. On medium fire, heat an 8-inch nonstick sauté tray. Using cooking spray to spray and include mushrooms and Spinach.

2. Sauté the Spinach and mushrooms for 2-3 minutes or before the spinach wilts.

3. If needed, whisk the egg and egg whites into a bowl of feta cheese and pepper. Pour the egg mixture into the pan over the vegetables.

4. Continue to cook the eggs for another 3-4 minutes while stirring with a spatula or until the eggs are cooked completely.

3.19 Steel Cut Oat Blueberry Pancakes

YIELD: 10 Servings

Ingredients

- ½ cup + 2 tablespoons of agave nectar

- ½ cup vanilla flavor Greek yogurt

- ½ cup of steel-cut oats

- ½ teaspoon of baking powder

- 1 cup blueberries (frozen)

- 1 cup of Milk

- 1 cup of whole wheat flour

- 1 egg

- 1/8 teaspoon of sea salt

- 1-1/2 cups of water

Directions:

1. Bring water to boil in a medium pot and add salt and steel-cut oats. Reduce the heat to a low simmer and cook for about 10 minutes until the oats are tender. Remove from the heat.

2.Combine the whole wheat pastry flour, baking powder, egg, baking soda, milk and yogurtin a medium mixing dish. Mix it to shapes a batter. Gently fold in the cooked oats and blueberries.

3. Heat a medium-heated grill rack or nonstick skillet and spray with cooking oil. Spoon a quarter cup of batter on the surface and cook until the pancakes start bubbling and are mildly brown. If necessary, operating in batches around 2-3 minutes per hand.

4. Garnish with around one tablespoon agave for each pancake

3.20 Cabbage And Dal Paratha

YIELD: 4 Servings

Ingredients

<u>For Dough</u>

- ½ cup of oats flour and ½ cup wheat flour

- ¼ tablespoon salt

<u>For Stuffing</u>

- ¼ cup of finely chopped mint leaves

- ¼ cup of soaked & boiled moong dal

- ¼ cup of finely chopped onions

- ¾ cup of finely chopped cabbage

- 1 pinch of turmeric powder

- 1 tablespoon fennel seeds

- 1 tablespoon grated ginger

- 1 tablespoon oil

- 1/8 tablespoon salt

- 2 tablespoons dry mango powder

- 2 tablespoon finely chopped green chilies

Directions:

<u>For Dough</u>

1. In a cup, combine the wheat flour, oatmeal and salt.

2. Add sufficient water to make a moist pastry.

3. For 3-4 minutes, knead the mixture very well and place it aside.

<u>For Stuffing</u>

1. Heat the oil in the pan first, then cook the fennel seeds.

2. Put the onions in sauté until golden brown.

3. Then add green chilies and cabbage and cook for a minute on a medium flame.

4. Put the mint leaves, dried mango powder, turmeric, and 1 tbsp of water to the moong dal. Mix and cook over a medium flame for 2 minutes.

5. Divide the mixture into five equal parts.

<u>Making Of Paratha</u>

1. Create five equal pieces of the dough

2. Roll the dough out in a circle,

3. In the middle of the rolled circle, put a part of the stuffing.

4. Start to get both sides together in the middle. Tightly seal it

5. By using a rolling pin, roll the stuffed dough into a circle again (for fast-rolling, sprinkle the wheat flour on a rolling base)

6. Use a preheated pan to cook both sides of the paratha until golden brown. Use the 1/4 tsp of oil.

7. Ready to feed, piping hot and nutrient-filled cabbage and dal paratha. Serve along with tomato chutney or mint.

3.21 Red Velvet Pancakes with Cream Cheese Topping

YIELD: 5 Servings

Ingredients

Cream Cheese Topping:

- 1 tablespoon milk (fat-free)

- 2 ounces 1/3 cream cheese (less fat)

- 3 tablespoons honey

- 3 tablespoons of plain yogurt (fat-free)

Pancakes:

- 2 ¼ teaspoons of baking powder

- 1 teaspoon vanilla

- 1 large egg

- 2 tablespoons + 1 cup milk (fat-free)

- ½ teaspoon food coloring (red paste)

- ½ tablespoon cocoa powder (unsweetened)

- ½ cup of whole wheat flour

- ½ cup all-purpose flour (unbleached)

- ¼ teaspoon of salt

- ¼ cup of sugar

Directions:

1. Mix and set aside the cream cheese coating ingredients.

2. In a large dish, combine the flour, baking powder, chocolate powder, sugar, and salt.

3. Dissolve the food coloring with the milk in another one; whisk in the egg and vanilla.

4. Take note not to overmix the wet and dry products until there are no longer dry spots.

5. On a medium-low fire, heat a large nonstick griddle pan. Spray lightly with oil to cover when wet, and spill 1/4 cup of the pancake batter into the pan.

6. Flip the pancakes as long as the pancake begins to bubble, and the edges start to settle. Repeat for the remaining batter.

7. Place 2 pancakes on each plate to eat, then finish with approximately 2-1/2 tablespoons of cream cheese topping.

3.22 Scrambled Eggs with Spinach

YIELD: 1 serving

Ingredients

- 2 Eggs

- 1 medium tomato (chopped)

- ½ teaspoon of cayenne pepper

- ½ teaspoon of fresh basil or cilantro or parsley

- ¼ cup of Swiss cheese

- 1 large handful of Spinach chopped

Directions:

1. Mix the chickens, basil and cayenne pepper in a large bowl. To beat until frothy, use a rotational beater or wire whisk.

2. Pour into a ready-made skillet. Start softly yet constantly stirring eggs immediately with a plastic or wooden spatula until the mixture resembles small fragments of fried egg covered by liquid egg. Add the tomatoes and Spinach.

3. Cook for an additional 30 to 60 seconds or until the egg is fixed but glossy.

4. Sprinkle with cheese (swiss) and new ground pepper.

5. Cover it with parsley.

6. Raise and fold one side of the omelet partly over the filling, using a spatula.

7. On a warm platter, arrange the remaining Spinach.

3.23 Tofu and Mushroom Scramble

YIELD: 3 servings

Ingredients

- A little lemon/lime juice

- ½ Avocado (ripe)

- 1 package of pressed tofu or extra-firm (crumbled)

- 1/2 diced red pepper

- 1/2 tablespoon of cumin, chili powder, garlic powder & chia seeds, pepper

- 1/4 cup of grated carrot

- 1/4 cup of diced red onion

- 2 cloves of garlic

- 2 Spring Onions (finely chopped)

- 4 large sliced white mushrooms

- Turmeric mixed with 3 tablespoons of water

Directions:

1. Over medium fire, heat a nonstick pan.

2. Add the garlic, red pepper, red onion, mushrooms and grated carrot and simmer for around 6 to 7 minutes before the onions and mushrooms start to soften.

3. When required, add a little water.

4. To the pan, add the crumbled tofu and spice mixture.

5. Stir well to mix it all up and fry before the tofu is cooked up.

6. Serve in a cup and finish with sliced avocado and scatter with spring onions and lemon or lime juice.

3.24 MUSHROOM and SAUSAGE QUICHE

YIELD: 2 servings

Ingredients

- ¼ cup of Swiss Cheese (grated)

- ¼ cup of sliced scallions

- ½ teaspoon of ground black pepper

- 1 cup of milk (1%)

- 1 teaspoon olive oil

- 3 egg whites

- 5 eggs

- 6 oz mushrooms

- 8 oz of turkey breakfast sausage with removed casing (cut into small pieces)

Directions:

1. Over medium-high heat, heat a large nonstick skillet. Add the sausage and cook for 6 to 8 minutes, until golden brown. Move it to a bowl for cooling.

2. To the pan, add oil. Add the mushrooms and cook, constantly stirring for 5 to 7 minutes, until golden brown. Transfer the mushrooms to the sausage bowl.

3. Leave for 5 minutes to cool. Stir in the scallions, pepper and cheese.

4. In a medium dish, whisk together the eggs, egg whites, and milk. Divide the egg mixture equally between the muffin cups that have been packed. Sprinkle the sausage mixture with a heaping tablespoon into each cup.

5. Place the rack in the middle of the oven; preheat to 325 °F. Kindly coat a nonstick muffin pan with cooking oil.

6. Bake until the tops tend to brown, for 25 minutes. Let it cool for 5 minutes on a wire rack. On top of the pan, place a plate, flip it over, and switch the quiches out off the rack. Turn upright

and let it cool.

3.25 Turmeric Milk

YIELD: 1 serving

Ingredients

- ½ teaspoon of turmeric powder

- ½ teaspoon of vanilla extract

- 1 tablespoon coconut oil

- 2 Cups of warm almond milk

Directions:

Blend or whisk until frothy and enjoy.

3.26 Poached Eggs with Avocado and Balsamic Tomatoes

YIELD: 2 servings

Ingredients

- 1 tablespoon of mixed Italian herbs or thyme

- 2 avocados

- 2 tablespoons of balsamic vinegar

- 2 tablespoons of olive oil

- per person 2 to 3 eggs

- 8 -10 tomatoes

Directions:

1. Put a pot of water to a boil (use sufficient water while the eggs are on the bottom to coat them). Directly smash the eggs into the boiling water, turn the heat down to mild for 2 minutes and then extract the product.

2. Chop up some tomatoes and cut the avocado while the eggs are frying. Use a spatula to separate the eggs from the water until the eggs are set.

3. Sprinkle with the Italian herbs, fresh herbs, and pepper; eat with fresh heirloom tomatoes, or roast with some balsamic vinegar if you have time.

3.27 Guacamole Deviled Eggs

YIELD: 3 servings

Ingredients

- 1 tablespoon of chives or green onion

- 1 tablespoon of Cilantro

- 1 tablespoon of Lime

- 1 tablespoon of Sour cream

- 1/2 chili pepper (jalapeno)

- 2 Avocados (ripe)

- 6 eggs (Hard Boiled) without shell and cut partially

Directions:

Add the ingredients in a bowl and mash with a yellow portion of an egg, slice the avocados, cut the pit and scoop the fruit out into a dish.

3.28 Pineapple Protein Smoothie

YIELD: 2 servings

Ingredients

- 2 tablespoon almond butter

- 2 dates (pitted)

- 2 tablespoon ground turmeric

- 1/2 cup of ice

- 3/4 cup of Milk

- 3/4 cup of pineapple chunks

- 3/4 cup of rinsed and drained canned chickpeas

Directions:

Mix all the ingredients until smooth.

3.29 Mixed Vegetable Thoran

YIELD: 2 servings

Ingredients

- ¼ cup of green peas

- ¼ tablespoon urad dal

- ½ cup of finely chopped carrots

- ½ cup of finely chopped French beans

- ½ cup of chopped onions

- ½ tablespoon chili powder

- ½ tablespoon mustard seeds

- ½ tablespoon roasted cumin seeds

- 1 tablespoon oil

- 1/8 tablespoon salt

- 2 Kashmiri red chilies

- 2 tablespoons crushed garlic

Directions:

1. Heat the oil and place the mustard seeds in a pan.

2. Put urad dal, red chilies and garlic and sauté on a medium flame for 1 min until the seeds start to crackle.

3. Then add onions, carrots, French beans, salt & peas and sauté on a medium flame for 2 minutes again.

4. Then apply 2 teaspoons of water and mix them well.

5. Cover the pan with a lid and cook the mixture for 5-6 minutes over medium heat. stir occasionally.

6. Then add chili powder, ground cumin seeds and mix well. On a medium flame, cook this mixture for 1 minute. Stir occasionally

7. Your tasty and high in health and low salt and the vegetable dish is ready to eat. Serve with Bajra/Jowar Rotis and even better with wheat Rotis (both are rich in potassium, which is important for lowering blood pressure).

Chapter 4 - Lunch Recipes

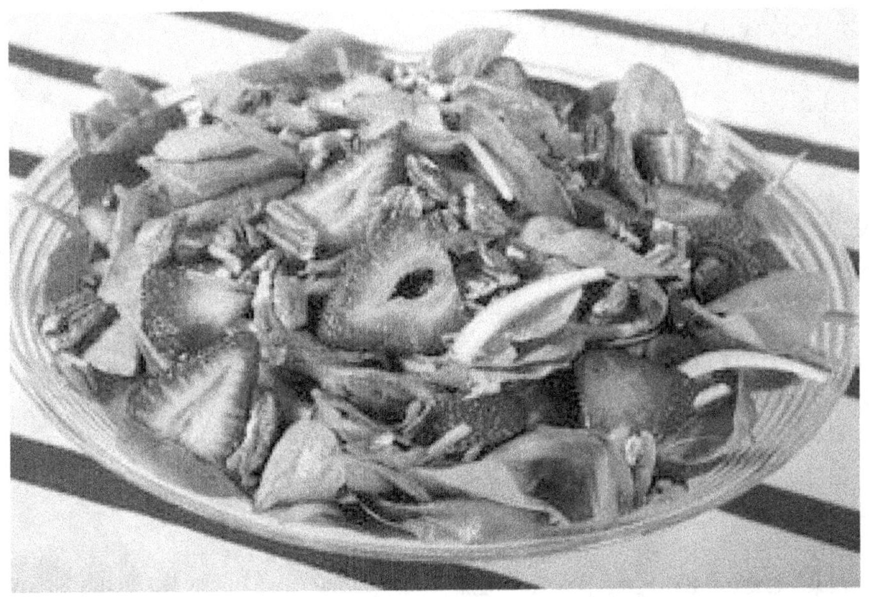

4.1 Quinoa Meatless Balls

YIELD: 24 servings

Ingredients

- 1 3/4 cup of grain bread crumbs

- 1 onion

- 1 tablespoon of olive oil (extra virgin)

- 1/2 tablespoon sea salt

- 1/3 cup of chives

- 1/3 cup of parmesan cheese

- 2 1/2 cup of cooked quinoa

- 3 cloves of garlic

- 4 eggs

Directions:

1. In a bowl, add all the ingredients and mix.

2.   Mix Mold into meatballs.

3.   The skillet is dipped with olive oil (extra virgin).

4.   Brown the meatballs for 10 minutes in a pan.

4.2 Quesadillas with Cilantro Yogurt Dip

YIELD: 4 Servings

Ingredients

- ½ finely chopped bell pepper

- ½ cup corn kernels

- ½ finely minced jalapeno pepper (optional)

- 1 cup of beans (black or pinto)

- 1 cup of low-fat cheese (shredded)

- 1 cup plain yogurt (nonfat)

- 1 medium carrot (shredded)

- 2 tablespoons cilantro (chopped)

- 2 Tablespoons cilantro (finely chopped)

- 6 corn tortillas (soft)

- Cilantro yogurt dip

- ½ of a lime Juice

Directions:

1. Over the low heat, preheat a large skillet.

2. Place 3 tortillas in rows. Divide the tortillas on cheese, rice, corn, cilantro, sliced carrots, and peppers.

3. With a second tortilla, cover each one.

4. Put a tortilla on the dry skillet and heat for about 3 minutes before the cheese melts, and the

tortilla is somewhat golden.

5. Flip and cook until golden from the other side, around 1 minute.

6. Mix the nonfat cream, lime juice and cilantro in a shallow dish.

4.3 Cauliflower Steak

YIELD: 2 SERVINGS

Ingredients

- ½ tablespoon of salt & pepper

- 1 head cauliflower

- 1 sprig chopped & stemmed thyme (fresh)

- 1 tablespoon chopped fresh rosemary

- 2 tablespoon olive oil (extra virgin)

- 3 minced cloves garlic

- 3 chopped sage leaves

- black pepper (fresh ground)

Directions:

1. Preheat to 400 °F in your oven. Remove the cauliflower leaves from the end of the stem, leaving the heart intact. Place the center side of the cauliflower down on a cutting board. Slice the cauliflower into four steaks from the middle of the cauliflower by using a large knife. Every steak should have a thickness of around a half-inch.

2. Put parchment paper on the baking sheet and use a teaspoon of olive oil to the top. On the baking dish, arrange the cauliflower steaks together with some of the split florets.

3. Combine most olive oil, chopped garlic, salt, pepper, and herbs in a separate dish. With this combination, spray the cauliflower slices evenly on both sides, but make sure the oil and herbs protect all the crevices.

4. Roast for 20 minutes in the oven. Flip the cauliflower and bake until golden brown and cooked

through for another 10 minutes.

5. Remove from the oven when the cauliflower steaks are cooked, and transfer to the individual serving plates. Season with the fresh ground black pepper in a generous amount.

4.4 Sunshine Wrap

YIELD: 4 Servings

Ingredients

- ¼ cup minced onion

- ¼ teaspoon of black pepper

- ¼ teaspoon of garlic powder

- ½ cup diced celery

- 1 large wheat tortilla (whole)

- 1 teaspoon of soy sauce

- 2 tablespoons of mayonnaise

- 2/3 cup of canned mandarin oranges (drained)

- 4 large washed & patted dry lettuce leaves

- 8 oz chicken breast piece (one large)

Directions:

1. In a nonstick pan, cook chicken breast on medium-high heat until the internal temperature hits the 165ºF. When the chicken has cooled enough to handle, cut into ½ inch cubes.

2. In a medium-sized bowl, mix the onions, oranges, chicken and celery. Add mayonnaise, garlic, pepper and soy sauce. Meld gently until chicken mixture is uniformly coated.

3. Put the tortilla on a neat cutting board or open plate. With a sharp knife or clean kitchen scissors, cut the tortilla into four quarters. Set 1 lettuce leaf on each tortilla quarter, trimming the leaf to hang over the tortilla.

4. Put one-fourth part of the chicken mixture in the center of every lettuce leaf. Roll up the tortillas into a cone shape, with the two edges getting together and the arched edge creating the cone's opening. Eat like a sandwich wrap.

5. Refrigerate leftovers within 2 hours.

7. Cut each quesadilla into 4 wedges (12 wedges total) and serve 3 wedges per person with about ¼ cup of the dip.

8. Refrigerate leftovers within 2 hours.

4.5 Southwest Style Rice Bowl

YIELD: 2 Servings

Ingredients

- 4 tablespoons of salsa
- 2 tablespoons of shredded cheese
- 2 tablespoons of sour cream (low fat)
- 1 teaspoon of vegetable oil
- 1 cup chopped or shredded cooked meat
- 1 cup brown rice (cooked)
- 1 cup vegetable mixture - onion bell peppers, zucchini, corn and tomato (chopped).

Directions:

1. Heat up the oil in a medium skillet over medium-high heat (in an electric skillet at 350 degrees Fahrenheit). Add the vegetables and cook for 3-5 minutes or until the vegetables are crisp and tender.

2. On the skillet, add cooked beef, tofu or beans and cooked rice and fire.

3. Split the rice mixture into two containers. Cover with cheese, sour cream & salsa and serve it warm.

4. Leftovers should be refrigerated within 2 hours.

4.6 Southwestern Black Bean Cakes with Guacamole

YIELD: 4 Servings

Ingredients

- ½ medium seeded & peeled avocado

- 1 (15-ounce) rinsed & drained low sodium black beans

- 1 (7-ounce) chipotle peppers (in adobo sauce)

- 1 large egg

- 1 plum tomato (small)

- 1 tablespoon of lime juice

- 1 teaspoon of ground cumin

- 2 cloves of garlic

- 2 slices of whole wheat bread (torn)

- 3 tablespoons of fresh cilantro

Directions:

1. In a food processor bowl or blender, put the broken bread. Cover and process or mix until coarse crumbs imitate the bread. Place the crumbs in a big bowl and set them aside.

2. Using cilantro and garlic to process or combine until finely chopped. Add 1 or 2 teaspoons of adobo sauce, rice, 1 chipotle pepper, and cumin. The mixture starts to pull away from the sides using on/off pulses to process or combine until the beans are coarsely sliced.

3. In a cup, add the mixture to the bread crumbs. Add the egg and mix thoroughly.

4. Shape the mixture into four 1/2-inch-thick patties. Grill these on a lightly oil uncovered grill rack directly on medium heat for about 8 to 10 minutes or until the patties are heated. Rotate once.

5. Similarly, to mash avocado in small cups. Stir in the lime juice. Season with salt and pepper. Serve with guacamole and tomato patties.

4.7 Pesto & Mozzarella Stuffed Portobello Mushroom Caps

YIELD: 1 Serving

Ingredients

- ¼ cup of shredded mozzarella cheese (low-fat)

- 1 small diced Roma tomato

- 2 mushroom caps (portobello)

- 2 tablespoons of pesto

Directions:

1. Clean the mushrooms by using a dry or moist rag. By twisting softly, remove the roots.

2. Divide the pesto uniformly between the 2 caps of the mushroom.

3. Cover with chopped and shredded tomatoes and cheese.

4. Bake in the oven at 400 °F for 15 minutes.

4.8 Mayo-less Tuna Salad

YIELD: 2 Servings

Ingredients

- black pepper

- 5 oz. light tuna in water (drained)

- 2 cups of arugula

- 1 tablespoon of red wine vinegar

- 1 tablespoon of shaved parmesan cheese (fresh)

- 1 tablespoon of olive oil (extra virgin)

- 1 cup of cooked pasta from 2 oz dry

- ¼ cup green onion tops (chopped)

Directions:

1. Toss the tuna with the oil, onion, vinegar, cooked pasta and arugula in a large bowl.

2. On two plates, divide and top with pepper and Parmesan.

3. Serve Instantly.

4.9 Washington Apple Turkey Gyro

YIELD: 6 Servings

Ingredients

- ½ cup of plain yogurt (low fat/fat-free)

- ½ pound cooked chicken breast/turkey (cut into thin strips)

- 1 cored apple, if possible Golden Delicious; (finely chopped or sliced),

- 1 cup onion (sliced)

- 1 cup of sweet green pepper (thinly sliced)

- 1 cup of sweet red pepper (thinly sliced)

- 1 tablespoon of vegetable oil

- 2 tablespoons of lemon juice

- 6 warmed pocket pita bread (whole wheat)

Directions:

1. Heat the oil in a large skillet over medium heat. Place the onion, peppers and lemon juice in the mixture and cook until tender. Mix in the apple turkey and cook until the turkey is heated. Simply remove from the heat.

2. Cover with some of the mixtures for each pita; drizzle with the yogurt. Serve it warm.

4.10 Fresh Shrimp Spring Rolls

YIELD: 6 Servings

Ingredients

- ½ medium cucumber (thinly sliced)

- ¾ cup cilantro (fresh)

- 1 ¼ pounds-20 ounces cooked shrimp (deveined & peeled)

- 1 cup shredded carrots

- 12 basil leaves

- 12 bibs of lettuce leaves

- 12 sheets of rice paper

Directions:

1. Clean the lettuce, basil, cilantro, carrots and cucumber, and make them ready.

2. For quick access, place all the vegetables and shrimp on the counter assembly-line style.

3. On a clean cutting board, put down a wet paper towel. Place one sheet of rice paper on a paper towel under warm water till it wets.

4. Layer 1 leaf of lettuce, 1 leaf of basil, 1 tablespoon of cilantro, cucumber and carrots on the rice paper that is nearest to you at the end. Begin gently rolling the rice paper over the vegetables like a burrito.

5. Place around 4 shrimp on the rice paper while the vegetables are covered. Continue to fold up the rice paper like a burrito until it's all rolled up, and do not forget to tuck in the ends.

6. Repeat the process before you make all 12 rolls. Serve them immediately.

4.11 Pear, Turkey and Cheese Sandwich

YIELD: 2 Servings

Ingredients

- 1 USA pear, cored and thinly sliced

- 1/4 cup shredded low-fat mozzarella cheese

- 2 slices (1 oz. each) reduced-sodium cooked or smoked turkey

- 2 tsp Dijon-style mustard

- Coarsely ground pepper

Directions:

1. Spread 1 teaspoon of mustard on each slice of bread. Place each slice of bread with one slice of turkey. Arrange the turkey pear slices and sprinkle each with 2 tablespoons of cheese. Sprinkle pepper over it.

2. Broil for 2 to 3 minutes by keeping 4 to 6 inches away from the heat or until turkey and pears become heated and cheese melts. Slice each sandwich in half and serve open face.

4.12 Spinach, Mushroom and Mozzarella Wraps

YIELD: 2 Servings

Ingredients

- ¼ cup 1-ounce part-skim mozzarella cheese (shredded)

- ½ pound trimmed & steamed fresh spinach/arugula

- 1 plum diced tomato

- 1 tablespoon of olive oil

- 1 teaspoon of minced garlic

- 2 whole wheat of 8-inch tortillas

- 8 oz. fresh sliced mushrooms (approximately 2 ½ cups)

Directions:

1. Preheat the furnace to 350 ⁰F. Heat 1 tablespoon olive oil over high heat in a saucepan. Add the single piece of garlic and mushrooms. Be vigilant as they turn red-brown, then turn and sauté until the second side becomes the same.

2. Spread layers of lettuce, mozzarella, cooked mushrooms and onion on each tortilla. Roll up and put in a finely oiled baking bowl, seam-side down. Bake until the cheese is melted and warm for about 10 minutes.

3. Slice each tortilla into quarters crosswise. Serve as desired at warm or room temperature.

4.13 Heartfelt Tuna Melt

YIELD: 4 Servings

Ingredients

- Salt & black pepper for taste

- 6 ounces drained white tuna (packed in water)

- 3 ounces grated Cheddar cheese (reduced-fat)

- 2 whole-wheat split English muffins

- 1/4 cup Russian (low fat) or Island salad dressing

- 1/4 cup onion (chopped)

- 1/3 cup celery (chopped)

Directions:

1. Preheat the broiler.

2. Put the salmon, celery, salad dressing and onion together. season with salt and pepper.

3. Toast half the English muffin. On the baking sheet, put split-side-up and cover each one with 1/4 of the tuna mixture. Broil for 2-3 minutes or until completely cooked.

4. Top with the cheese and return to the broiler for about 1 minute before the cheese is melted.

4.14 Apple-Swiss Panini

YIELD: 4 Servings

Ingredients

- ¼ cup of honey mustard (nonfat)

- 1 cup of arugula leaves

- 2 thinly sliced crisp apples,

- 6 ounces thinly sliced Swiss cheese (low-fat)

- 8 slices of whole-grain bread

- Cooking spray

Directions:

1. On medium-heat, Preheat the panini press. Use just a nonstick skillet if you don't have a panini press.

2. Apply the honey mustard, gently and uniformly over each bread slice. Layer four slices of bread with apple slices, butter, and arugula leaves. Top each one with the remaining slices of bread.

3. Lightly coat the cooking spray with the panini press. Grill every sandwich for about 3 to 5 mins or until it is melted with cheese and toasted with bread. Remove from the pan before serving and let it to cool slightly.

4.15 California Grilled Veggie Sandwich

YIELD: 4 Servings

Ingredients

- ½ cup crumbled feta cheese (reduced-fat)

- 1 cup of sliced red bell peppers

- 1 sliced red onion

- 1 sliced small yellow squash

- 1 small sliced zucchini

- 1 tablespoon of lemon juice

- 1/8 cup of olive oil

- 2 slices of focaccia bread

- 3 cloves garlic (minced)

- 3 tablespoons of light mayonnaise

Directions:

1. Meld the mayonnaise, minced garlic, and lemon juice in a cup. Keep it in the refrigerator.

2. Preheat the grill to a high degree.

3. Brush the vegetables with olive oil. Brush the barbecue grill with oil. Place the bell peppers and zucchini nearest to the center of the grill and place bits of onion and squash around them. Cook for 3 minutes, turn and cook for 3 more minutes. It will take much longer for the peppers. Remove and set aside from the barbecue.

4. On the crust's cut sides, scatter some of the mayonnaise mixtures; sprinkle all with the feta cheese. Put on the grill in cheese side up position, and cover for 2 to 3 min with the lid. Carefully watch it so as not to burn the bottoms.

5. Take the bread from the grill and layer the vegetables with it. Enjoy the open-faced grilled sandwiches.

4.16 Terrific Tortellini Salad

YIELD: 8 main-dish Servings

Ingredients

- Milk (optional)

- 3 cups of broccoli florets

- 1/4 cup green onions (sliced)

- 1/2 cup bottled ranch salad dressing (reduced-fat)

- 1 large tomato (chopped)

- 1 cup of fresh pea pods (halved)

- 1 cup of crinkle-cut/sliced carrots - 2 medium

- 1 9-ounce package of refrigerated light cheese tortellini/ravioli

Directions:

1. Cook the pasta according to product instructions in a large saucepan. During the last 3 minutes of preparation, add the broccoli and carrots. Drain it. Rinse with some cold water. Again drain it.

2. Mix the cooked pasta mixture and green onions in a large bowl; sprinkle with dressing. To coat, toss softly. For 2 to 24 hours, cover it and then cool.

3. Stir the tomato and pea pods gently into the pasta mixture before eating. To moisten, stir in a little milk if necessary. For serving, make eight main-dishes.

4.17 Tuscan-Style Tuna Salad

YIELD: 4 (1 cup each) Servings

Ingredients

- 1 15-ounce can of small white beans like cannellini/great northern (rinsed)

- 1/4 teaspoon salt

- 10 cherry tomatoes (quartered)

- 2 6-ounce cans of chunk light tuna (drained)

- 2 tablespoons of olive oil (extra-virgin)

- 2 tablespoons of lemon juice

- 4 scallions (trimmed & sliced)

- Freshly ground pepper for taste

Directions:

1. In a medium dish, combine the fish, beans, onions, oil, scallions, lemon juice, pepper, and

salt.

2. Stir it slowly. Refrigerate until it is ready.

4.18 Strawberry, Melon & Avocado Salad

YIELD: 4 Servings

Ingredients

- 1 1/2 cups sliced hulled strawberries

- 1 small avocado 4-5 ounces (peeled up, pitted and cut into 16 slices)

- 1/4 cup honey

- 1/4 teaspoon ground pepper (fresh)

- 16 slices of about 1/2 small cantaloupe (thin & rind removed)

- 2 tablespoons fresh mint (finely chopped)

- 2 tablespoons of sherry vinegar/red-wine vinegar

- 2 teaspoons toasted sesame seeds

- 4 cups of baby spinach

- Pinch of salt

Directions:

1. In a small cup, whisk the honey, mint, vinegar, pepper and salt.

2. Divide the Spinach into 4 plates of lettuce. On top of the Spinach, place alternating pieces of cantaloupe and avocado. Top the strawberries for each salad, sprinkle with dressing and scatter with the sesame seeds.

4.19 Roast Chicken Dal

YIELD: 4 (1 1/2 cups each) Servings

Ingredients

- 1 1/2 teaspoons of canola oil

- 1 14-ounce canned tomatoes (diced & preferably fire-roasted)

- 1 15-ounce lentil Can (rinsed) or 2 cups of cooked lentils

- 1 2-pound of roasted chicken with discarded skin, meat separated from bones & diced (4 cups)

- 1 small onion (minced)

- 1/4 cup plain yogurt (low-fat)

- 1/4 teaspoon salt for taste

- 2 teaspoons of curry powder

Directions:

1. Heat oil over medium to high heat heavy saucepan. Include the onion and fry, stirring for 3 to 4 minutes, until tender but not browned.

2. Add the curry powder and simmer for 20 to 30 seconds, stirring until mixed with the onion and deep aromatics.

3. Whisk in lentils, tomatoes, salt and chicken and cook until it is heated fully, stirring regularly.

4. Turn off the heat and apply the yogurt, and stir. Serve it instantly.

4.20 Spaghetti Squash with Chunky Tomato Sauce

YIELD: 6 Servings

Ingredients

- 1 pound of lean ground beef

- 2 cloves of minced garlic

- 2 tablespoons of tomato paste

- 1 recipe Cooked Spaghetti Squash

- Small & fresh basil leaves

- 1 14 1/2-ounce Canned tomatoes (diced & undrained)

- 1/2 cup 1 medium onion (chopped)

- 1/2 cup 1 small green sweet pepper (chopped)

- 1-1/2 teaspoons crushed Italian seasoning (dried)

- 1/4 cup 1-ounce Parmesan cheese (shredded)

- 1 8-ounce tomato sauce Can

- 1/8 teaspoon of black pepper

Directions:

1. Cook the ground beef, sweet pepper onion, and garlic in a wide saucepan until the meat is brown. Drain it. Add the diced and undrained tomatoes, black pepper tomato sauce, tomato paste, and Italian seasoning. Boil the sauce and minimize the heat. Simmer and uncovered for 15 minutes and stir for some time.

2. Meanwhile, cooking of the Spaghetti Squash. Serve the sauce over squash. Sprinkle the cheese with Parmesan. Garnish with basil leaves if needed.

3. Cooked Spaghetti Squash: In many spots, a sharp knife pokes a 2-1/2 - 3-pound whole spaghetti squash. Put the squash in a microwave-safe baking dish. Microwave the uncovered for 10 to 15 minutes on 100 percent (high) capacity or until tender. Let wait for five minutes. Halve the thickness of the squash and cut the seeds. Shred and split the squash pulp into strands using two forks. Make 6 parts for serving.

Chapter 5 – Dinner

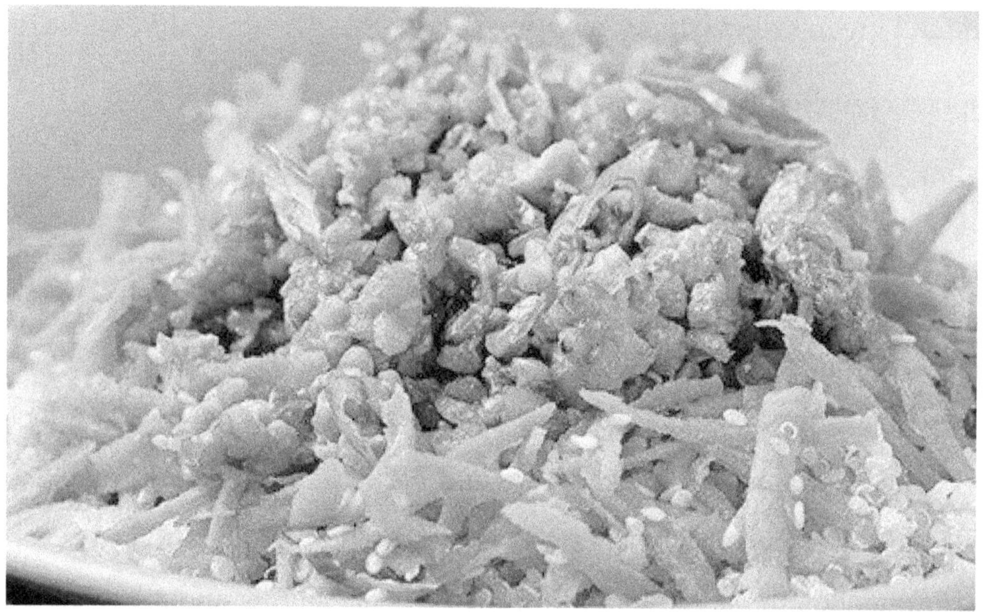

5.1 Meatier Meatloaf

YIELD: 6 servings

Ingredients

- 6 oz. of white mushrooms (trimmed & thinly sliced)

- 3/4 pepper

- 3 tablespoons with 1/2 cup chicken broth (low-sodium)

- 3 tablespoons of packed brown sugar

- 2 tablespoons of Dijon mustard

- 2 tablespoons of unsalted butter

- 2 tablespoons of soy sauce

- 2 large eggs

- 2 minced garlic cloves

- 1/4 cup of cider vinegar

- 1/3 cup fresh parsley (minced)

- 1/2 tablespoon of ground coriander

- 1/2 tablespoon of dried thyme

- 1/2 slice of white sandwich bread (split into 1" piece)

- 1/2 cup of ketchup

- 1 tablespoon of hot sauce

- 1 tablespoon of unflavored gelatin

- 1 tablespoon of tomato paste

- 1 onion (chopped & fine)

- 1-pound ground pork

- 1-pound lean ground beef (85%)

Directions:

1. For the meatloaf: Change the oven rack's center location and fire the oven to 350 degrees Fahrenheit. Fold heavy-duty aluminum foil into a 5-inch rectangle to form 9. Cover the foil in a rimmed baking sheet mounted on a wire shelf. Poke holes with a skewer (approximately 1/2 inch apart) in the foil. Spray the foil with a spray of vegetable oil.

2. In a 12-inch skillet over medium heat, melt the butter. Add the onion and mushrooms; fry and stirring regularly for 10 to 12 minutes, until the color is brown. Add the tomato paste and simmer for about 3 minutes and mix continuously, until browned. Reduce heat to low and add 3 tablespoons of broth and garlic. Cook to remove any browned pieces, scraping the plate's bottom until thickened, for around 1 minute. To cool, shift the mushroom mixture to a wide dish.

3. Whisk together the eggs, the remaining half a cup of broth, and the soy sauce in a bowl. Sprinkle the gelatin over the egg mixture and leave to rest for about 5 minutes until the gelatin softens.

4. Pulse the bread until finely ground in the food processor at 5 to 10 pulses. To bread-crumbs, add gelatin blend, cooled mushroom blend, mustard, parsley, thyme and pepper. And pulse them until the mushrooms are finely ground, around 10 pulses, scraping down the bowl as desired. Place the bread-crumb mixture in a wide dish. To fully blend, add pork and beef and meld with

your hands.

5. Move the meat mixture to the rectangle foil and use wet hands to create a 9 by 5-inch loaf. Bake the meatloaf for 75 to 90 minutes until the heat reaches 155 to 160 degrees Fahrenheit. Take the broiler from the oven and turn it on.

6. For the glaze: When the meatloaf is frying, put all the ingredients in a small saucepan over medium heat to boil. Cook and stirring regularly for about 5 minutes, until it becomes thick and syrupy.

7. Spread half of the glaze uniformly over the cooked meatloaf; put under the broiler and cook for around 2 minutes before the glaze bubbles and starts browning at the edges. Remove the meatloaf from the oven and cover thinly with the remaining glaze. Return to the broiler and cook for about 2 minutes longer before the glaze bursts again and starts to brown. Before slicing and serving, let the meatloaf cool for 20 minutes.

5.2 Salmon With Broccoli & Red Potatoes

YIELD: 2 servings

Ingredients

- 1 tablespoon whole-grain mustard

- 1 tablespoon lemon juice

- 1 tablespoon along with 2 tablespoon olive oil (extra virgin)

- 1/2-pound broccoli florets (torn into 2" pieces)

- 1/2-pound small red potatoes (unpeeled & halved)

- 1/2 tablespoon honey

- 2 (6oz-8oz) of center-cut without salmon fillets(1 - 1 ½" thick)

- 2 tablespoon fresh minced chives

- salt & ground black pepper for taste

Directions:

1. Set the lowest location of the toaster oven rack, pick the convection setting, and heat the oven to 500 °F.

2. Clean all over with 1 teaspoon oil and spray with 1/4 teaspoon salt and 1/4 teaspoon pepper. Dry with paper towels. Until required, refrigerate it.

3. Brush the rimmed baking sheet, with a 1 tablespoon oil toaster oven. Apply 1/2 tablespoon of oil to the potatoes, season with salt & pepper, and place the cut side down on half of the pan.

4. Apply 1/2 tablespoon of oil to the broccoli, season with salt and pepper and place on the other half of the board. Heat until potatoes are light golden brown and broccoli on the bottom is dark brown for 22 to 24 minutes, rotating the sheet halfway while baking.

5. Meanwhile, mix the chives, mustard, honey, lemon juice, 1 tablespoon of oil left in the bowl, and make a season with the salt and pepper.

6. Keep it warm, take the sheet from the oven, and pass the bowl's broccoli. To make it browned, cover with foil. Remove any pieces of broccoli left on the sheet by using a spatula. Keep the potatoes on the pan.

7. Place the salmon skin side down on the mat and spread equally. Place the sheet in the oven and reduce the temperature of the oven to 275 °F instantly. Bake until the fillet centers reaches at 125 °F (medium-rare) for 11 to 15 minutes, turning the sheet halfway through the baking process. Move the potatoes and salmon to your broccoli platter. Serve with a dressing of chives.

5.3 Daphne Oz's Stuffed Peppers

YIELD: 3 servings

Ingredients

- 1 cup cooked wild rice, grains, quinoa & farro

- 1 tablespoon of chile powder

- 1 tablespoon of cumin

- 1/2 cup of black beans

- 1/2 cup of grated jack cheese

- 1/2-pound ground turkey

- 1-2 cups grilled veggies such as zucchini and onion (diced)

- 2 cloves minced garlic

- 3 poblano peppers (half cut & with removed seeds)

- 3 tablespoons of olive oil (divided)

- Greek yogurt (optional)

- Kosher salt and cracked black pepper, to taste

- lime wedges (optional)

- salsa (optional)

- sliced avocado (optional)

Directions:

1. First, heat the oven to 375 °F.

2. On a sheet pan lined with parchment, put the peppers and sprinkle with the olive oil and season with pepper and salt.

3. Place them in the oven and cook until tender for 15-18 minutes, but they should still retain their form. Take it out of the oven and set it aside.

4. Over a medium-high flame, heat a large skillet and add the remaining olive oil. To the pan, add the ground turkey, season with pepper and salt and all the spices. Add the garlic and cook for about five more minutes before the turkey has been browned. Remove and transfer to a wide bowl from the heat. Stir in the quinoa or the other grains, veggies, and beans on the barbecue. Taste and uniformly distribute the mixture between the peppers for seasoning.

5. Top with the cheese and put it back in the oven for another 15 minutes until the cheese melts and the entire filling is hot. On a plate, put each pepper and top with your favorite toppings.

5.4 Whole Grain Pasta & Pumpkin Bake

YIELD: 4 servings

Ingredients

- Kosher salt & cracked black pepper for taste

- 3/4-pound whole-grain penne

- 1/2 tablespoon paprika

- 1 cup toasted whole wheat bread-crumbs

- 1 clove garlic (peeled)

- 1 (15 oz)-Can of pumpkin puree (unsweetened)

- 1 (15 oz)-Can of coconut milk

Directions

1. First, heat the oven to 350°F.

2. Put a big pot to boil the water and season with salt liberally. Following the package directions, cook the pasta for 2 minutes. Reserve and set aside 2 cups of pasta water. Drain the spaghetti, put it in a mixing bowl and set it aside.

3. In a mixer, mix the coconut milk, ginger, pumpkin puree, salt and plenty of crushed black pepper. Blend until smooth, and add (if necessary) some pasta water to make it thin. The noodles drain a lot of the sauce, so it should be thin enough to easily pour from the carafe.

4. Pour over the spaghetti with the pumpkin sauce and stir to coat. Cover with bread-crumbs and put in a baking dish. Place for 15 minutes in the oven until golden brown color appears, bubbling along the edges.

5.5 Daphne Oz's Philly Cheesesteak Tacos

YIELD: 4 servings

Ingredients

- 5 button mushrooms/creminis (stemmed by caps-thinly sliced)

- 4-6 6" flour tortillas

- 2 tablespoon butter (unsalted)

- 2 tablespoon olive oil (extra virgin)

- 2 oregano sprigs/1 teaspoon dried

- 1 teaspoon of Kosher salt

- 1 thinly sliced, cored & seeded red bell pepper

- 1 lb. skirt steak

- 1 halved & thinly sliced medium onion

- 1 cup of low-moisture mozzarella/Monterey jack cheese

Directions:

1. Melt butter over medium heat in a medium skillet. Season with salt and pepper on the steak, and transfer to the pan. For medium-rare or longer, sear on both sides for 4 minutes if you want it to cook more. Take the steak out of the pan and let it sit for 10 minutes.

2. Cover the pan with 1 teaspoon of olive oil and add the oregano and onion. To caramelize the onions, simmer for 30 minutes over a low flame. Stir in the bell peppers and simmer for about 5 more minutes until they become soft.

3. Take the steak out of the pan and apply the remaining olive oil along with the mushrooms to the pan. Cook until browned and introduce salt to the seasoning.

4. Cut the steak with the mushrooms and add them to the pan. Stir in the peppers and onions. Top with the cheese and to melt, cover the plate.

5. Heat the tortillas and fill with the top. Now you can serve.

5.6 Vegetables and Turkey Stir-Fry

YIELD: 8 Servings

Ingredients

- Thin slices & minced ginger root

- 3 cups cooked brown rice

- 2 cups chopped fresh, canned or frozen vegetables such as mushrooms, bok choy, celery & water chestnuts

- 1 tablespoon oil

- 1 cup turkey (cut into ½" cubes)

- 1 peeled & minced clove garlic/1/8 tsp garlic powder

- ½ teaspoon sugar

- ½ teaspoon salt

Directions:

1. Heat the oil over medium heat in a large skillet. Add the salt, the turkey, the root of ginger, the garlic, and the vegetables. For 1 minute, please do a stir-fry. To avoid scorching, reduce the heat. Only add sugar.

2. Remove the pan from the heat until the vegetables are tender. Add 1-2 tablespoons of water and simmer for 2 more minutes until tender or if the vegetables are still hard. Serve with rice (or noodles). Leftovers can be refrigerated within 2-3 hours.

5.7 Pantry Minestrone

YIELD: 8 servings

Ingredients

- Kosher salt & cracked black pepper for taste

- 6 cups vegetable /chicken stock (low-sodium)

- 3 tablespoons of basil pesto

- 2 tablespoons of tomato paste

- 2 tablespoons of olive oil

- 2 cups frozen (thawed) vegetable medley

- 2 cups frozen (thawed) broccoli

- 2 cloves sliced garlic

- 2 drained & rinsed-Can of white beans

- 1 sweet potato (peeled & diced)

- 1 onion (diced)

- 1 cup Spinach (frozen)

- 1 bay leaf

- 1 (28 oz) can of whole peeled tomatoes (roughly chopped)

Directions:

1. Over medium to high heat, warm up a big Dutch oven or soup pot and add olive oil. Add the onions, garlic, sweet potatoes, and season with salt and pepper when warmed.

2. Add the tomato paste and simmer for an extra 3 minutes. Add the broccoli, Spinach and veggies and cook until it gets warm. Boil and stir in the tomatoes, beans, and stock. Put the bay leaf in and reduce the heat to a low level.

3. For 25 to 30 minutes, cook. Taste and ladle into bowls for seasoning. Using basil pesto for topping and serve with crusty bread.

5.8 Tex-Mex Loaded Baked Sweet Potatoes

YIELD: 4 Servings

Ingredients

- ¼ cup cilantro or scallions (chopped)

- ½ cup Greek yogurt / light sour cream (fat-free)

- ½ cup Mexican cheese blend (reduced fat)

- ½ cup salsa (non-compulsory)

- ½ red onion (diced about ½ cup)

- ½ teaspoon cumin

- ½ teaspoon paprika

- 1 1/3 cups of canned sodium black beans (reduced, rinsed and drained)

- 1 red pepper (diced about ½ cup)

- 1 teaspoon of chili powder

- 1 teaspoon of low sodium taco seasoning

- 1 teaspoon of olive oil

- 4 medium-sized potatoes (sweet)

- Pinch of salt

Directions:

1. Poke holes with a fork in the potato, cook on the potato setting of your microwave until the potatoes are soft and cooked through (for 4 potatoes, around 8-10 minutes on high). Cook in the oven for around 45 minutes at 400 °F, if you don't have a microwave.

2. In a shallow bowl, add the yogurt and taco seasoning and meld well.

3. Heat oil over low heat in a medium pot. Add the peppers, chili powder, onions, paprika, salt and cumin and simmer for around 5 minutes until the onions are gently caramelized.

4. Now include black beans and mix to blend and heat (approximately for 5 more minutes).

5. Cut down the potato lengthwise or use a fork to pierce the surface.

6. Cover with 1/3 cup of black bean blend, 2 tablespoons of shredded cheese, 2 tablespoons of Greek yogurt blend and 2 tablespoons of salsa.

5.9 Tandoori Chicken

YIELD: 6 Servings

Ingredients

- 6 boneless, skinless chicken breasts (cut into 1-2" pieces)

- 6 skewers (soaked in water, at least for 15 minutes)

- 5 crushed garlic cloves

- 2 tablespoon paprika

- 1 teaspoon yellow curry powder

- 1 teaspoon ground ginger

- 1 teaspoon red pepper flakes - crushed (use ½ teaspoon for a milder flavor)

- 1 cup plain yogurt (nonfat)

- ½ cup lemonade

Directions:

1. 1st heat the oven to 400 °F. In a blender, combine the milk, garlic, lemon juice, ginger, yellow curry powder, red pepper flakes and paprika and mix smoothly.

2. Onto each of the soaked skewers, skewer the equivalent number of chicken bits. Place the chicken skewers in a shallow casserole dish. Add half of a mixture of yogurt, and reserved the rest. Cover for about 15 minutes and cool.

3. With cooking sauce, spray another small baking dish. Remove the chicken skewers, dispose of the marinade with the yogurt, and put the chicken skewers in the bowl. Brush the chicken with a blend of reserved yogurt.

4. Bake for 15-20 minutes or until juices run clear when meat is pierced. Instantly serve. Grill the chicken, skewers over medium-high heat for 3-5 minutes on either hand for much more authentic preparation.

5.10 Turkey Fajitas Bowls

YIELD: 4 Servings

Ingredients

- 4 tablespoons salsa (for topping)

- 4- 8 inches corn tortillas (or you can make your particular tostada bowls)

- 3/4 tsp fresh chile pepper or dried for taste

- 2 tsp olive oil

- 1/2 tsp dried oregano leaves

- 1/2 lb. turkey breast

- 1/2 large piece yellow bell pepper (cut into 1" piece)

- 1/2 big green pepper (cut into 1" piece)

- 1/2 cup cheddar cheese (shredded) for topping

- 1 tbsp lemon juice

- 1 medium tomato (pierce into 12 wedges)

- 1 crushed clove Garlic

Directions:

1. Tear the turkey into thin slices and then into 3/4-inch short strips. Add 1 tablespoon of oil with garlic, lemon juice, oregano and chili pepper in a medium dish. Add the turkey and stir for coating. Let it marinate for half an hour.

2. Heat the remaining 1 tbsp oil in a nonstick skillet at medium-high heat. Stir in the yellow and green peppers and fry for 2 minutes. Add the turkey strips and fry for an extra 3 minutes. Heat the tomatoes and stir.

3. In a pan, hot tortillas are used as a basis. Pour in the bowl of tortilla or tostada and top with salsa and cheese.

5.11 Sesame-Honey Chicken & Quinoa Bowl

YIELD: 4 Servings

Ingredients

Quinoa and carrot slaw:

- 3/4 cup quinoa, rinsed

- 1 & 1/2 cup water

- 2 cups of grated carrots (approximately 3 large)

- 2 tbsp rice vinegar

- 2 tbsp toasted sesame seeds

- 1 tbsp sesame oil

Sesame-Honey Chicken:

- 3 tablespoons reduced-sodium soy sauce

- 3 tablespoons honey

- 2 tablespoons water

- 2 tbsp sesame oil

- 2 scallions (sliced)

- 2 cups prepared chicken breast (pierce into the bite-sized pieces)

- 1 teaspoon cornstarch

Directions:

1. To make the quinoa: Boil 1½ cups of water in a shallow saucepan. Add the quinoa and put it to a boil again. Reduce to a medium boil, cover and cook for 10 to 14 minutes before the water is absorbed. Uncover them and wait.

2. Meanwhile, in a medium dish, mix the rice vinegar, carrots, rice vinegar, seeds, sesame and 1 tablespoon of the oil. Put it aside.

3. Combine the soy sauce, sesame oil, sugar, and cornstarch 2 teaspoons of water in a shallow cup. Pour it into a medium skillet. Cook and stir over medium heat until the sauce becomes thickened. Add the chicken and stir for about 1 minute before it is coated with the sauce.

4. Divide the quinoa and top each with 1/2 cup of carrot slaw and 3/4 cup of chicken mixture in 4 cups. Sprinkle with green onion.

5.12 Southwest Tortilla Bake

YIELD: 4 Servings

Ingredients

- Salsa

- Eight corn tortillas (cut in half)

- 3 eggs

- 2 green onions (sliced)

- 1/2 tsp chili powder

- 1 tomato (sliced)

- 1 cup Monterey Jack cheese (shredded)

- 1 cup fresh / frozen corn

- 1 cup milk (fat-free)

- 1 cup of cooked black / pinto beans

- 1 4-ounce can green chilies (diced)

Directions:

1. 1st heat the oven up to 350 °F.

2. Using nonstick spray or oil to coat an 8-inch square baking dish. Arrange 5 tortilla halves to line the bottom of the plate. Top each of cheese, corn and beans with 1/3 of a cup. Utilize 1/2 of the green onions to sprinkle. To layer and top with beans, 1/3 cup cheese, the leftover corn, and green onions, place a further 5 tortilla halves on top. To shield, place the last 5 tortilla pieces over the corner.

3. Add the eggs, chili powder and milk to a medium bowl and whisk to mix. Stir in the chilies. Pour the egg and milk mixture equally over the tortillas. Top with both the 1/3 cup of left cheese and tomato slices.

4. Uncovered and bake for about 50 minutes until a knife inserted in the middle. Let it stand at

room temperature for 10 minutes before serving. Serve hot with salsa.

5.13 Quick Chili

YIELD: 7 Servings

Ingredients

- 1 15.5-ounces-Can of kidney beans (drained)

- 1 14.5 ounces-Can of tomatoes with liquid (diced)

- 1/2-pound lean ground meat

- 1/2 medium onion (chopped)

- 1 1/2 tbsp chili powder

Directions:

1. Over medium-high heat, onions and brown meat in a large skillet (350 degrees Fahrenheit in an electric skillet). Drain the fat.

2. Add beans, chili powder and tomatoes.

3. Reduce the heat to low (in an electric skillet at 250 degrees Fahrenheit), cover and simmer for 10 minutes.

4. Serve it hot.

5. Leftovers can be refrigerated within 2-3 hours.

5.14 Sesame Encrusted Baked Chicken Tenders

YIELD: 4 Servings

Ingredients

- olive oil spray

- 6 tablespoons sesame seeds (toasted)

- 4 tbsp panko bread-crumbs (without adding the salt)

- 2 tsp sesame oil

- 2 teaspoons soy sauce (low sodium)

- 16-ounces chicken tenderloins

- ½ tsp coarse salt

Directions:

1. Preheat to above 425 degrees Fahrenheit and spray with parchment paper or nonstick oil spray on a baking sheet.

2. In a dish, mix the soy sauce and sesame oil. In another dish, combine the panko, sesame seeds and salt.

3. Put the chicken with the soy sauce and oil in the dish, then in the mixture with sesame seeds to coat properly.

4. Place this on the baking sheet and gently spray with oil spray on the top of the chicken and bake for 8-10 minutes. Switch over and simmer for 4-5 more minutes or until it is cooked through.

5.15 Shepherd's Pie

YIELD: 6 Servings

Ingredients

- 2 bulky baking potatoes (peeled & diced)

- 1 lb. lean ground beef

- 1 medium onion (chopped)

- 1 clove garlic (minced)

- ½ cup & 2 tablespoons flour

- 4 cups of frozen vegetables (mixed)

- ground pepper for taste

- 1/2 cup milk (low-fat)

- 1/2 cup cheddar cheese (shredded)

- 3/4 cup beef broth (reduced sodium)

Directions:

1. In a saucepan, put the diced potatoes and add enough water to barely cover. Just bring it to a boil. Diminish the heat and simmer, and covered it until soft (around 15 minutes).

2. Drain and mash the potatoes. Add milk and set aside the mixture.

3. Preheat the oven to 375 °C.

4. Put brown meat, garlic and onion in a large skillet. Stir in the flour. Cook and constantly stir for 1 minute.

5. Add the broth and vegetables. Cook for five minutes until it's bubbly. Just stir well.

6. Spoon the mixture of vegetables into an 8-inch square baking dish. Spread the mixture of potatoes over the vegetable/meat mixture. Sprinkle the cheese.

7. Bake for 25 minutes, until bubbly and hot.

8. Within 2-3 hours, refrigerate the leftovers.

Chapter 6 – Dessert

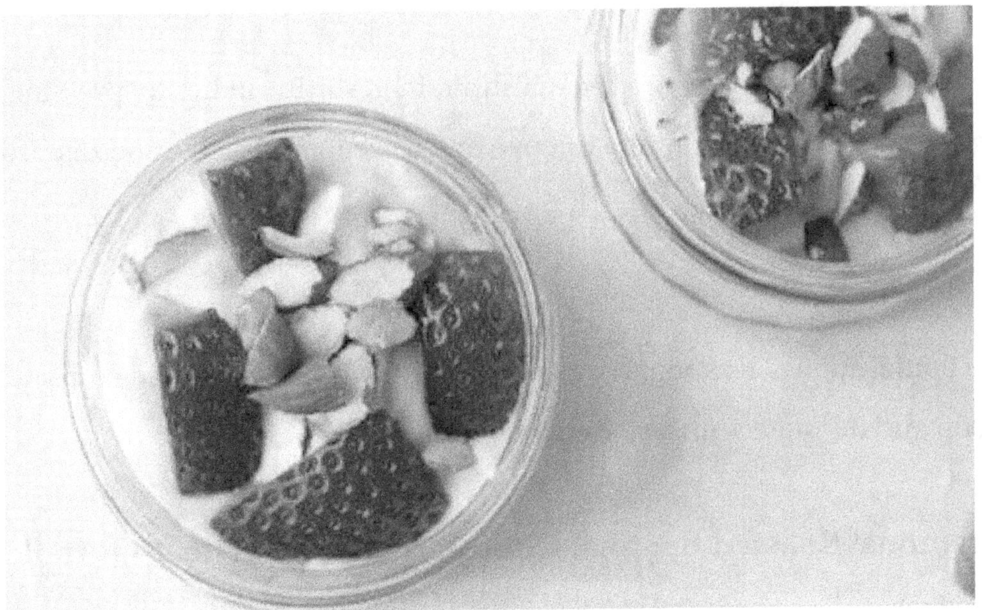

6.1 Gail Simmons' Cherry Vanilla Float

YIELD: 2 servings

Ingredients

- club soda/seltzer (chilled)

- vanilla ice cream

- whole frozen (thawed) pitted cherries for serving

- 2-1/2 cups of frozen dark cherries (pitted & finely chopped)

- 1/2 teaspoon crudely ground black pepper

- 2 tablespoon sugar

- 1/8 teaspoon pure vanilla extract

Directions

For the syrup:

1. In a shallow saucepan, combine the sliced cherries, cinnamon, pepper, salt and 3/4 of a water cup.

2. Bring over medium heat to an active boil and cook until it has a dense syrup consistency (around 15 minutes).

3. Strain the syrup into a bowl using a fine-mesh strainer, softly but tightly pressing on the solids and scraping the strainer's bottom to remove much syrup as feasible and discard the solids.

4. Stir in vanilla and cool thoroughly for 15 to 20 minutes. Makes 2/3 of a cup.

To make the float:

In an 8-ounce bottle, apply 2 teaspoons syrup and finish with 1/2 cup cold club soda. Attach an ice cream scoop and decorate with a few entire cherries.

6.2 Gail Simmons' Roasted Banana, Chocolate, Whole Wheat-Quinoa Bread

YIELD: 10 servings

Ingredients

- 1 teaspoon baking soda

- 2 tablespoon sugar

- 2 large eggs

- 4 bananas (3 coarsely mashed & 1 thin sliced lengthwise)

- 2 tablespoon yogurt

- 1 teaspoon pure vanilla extract

- 1/2 teaspoon cinnamon

- 1/2 cup of vegetable oil (for greasing pan)

- 1/2 cup of dark chocolate chips

- 1/4 teaspoon Kosher salt

- 3/4 cup and tablespoon whole wheat flour

- 3/4 cup of quinoa flour

Directions:

1. Preheat the oven to 350 degrees Fahrenheit. Oil a loaf pan generously, then sprinkle with 2 teaspoons of whole wheat flour and remove the extra flour.

2. Whisk together the whole wheat, baking soda, quinoa flour, cinnamon and salt in a bowl.

3. Whisk the sugar and eggs together in a separate bowl until smooth. In a slow stream, add milk, whisk until combined, then mix in the mashed bananas, vanilla and yogurt. Fold gently in the combination of flour and chocolate to mix.

4. In the prepared loaf pan, add the batter and finish with the remaining banana slices.

5. Bake for about 45 minutes until the bread becomes golden and then inject the wooden skewer in the middle to clean.

6. Cool the loaf for about 10 minutes in a pan on a wire rack, then switch on the rack. Turn the right side of the loaf up to allow slightly more cooling before slicing. Serve at room temperature or warm.

6.3 Heart Healthy Chocolate Chip Cookies

YIELD: 24 SERVINGS

Ingredients

- 4 tablespoon butter substitute
- 2 cups of rolled oats
- 1/4 teaspoon baking soda
- 1/3 cup dried cranberries
- 1/2 teaspoon salt
- 1/2 cup tahini
- 1/2 cup walnuts (chopped)
- 1 large egg
- 1 cup cacao chocolate chips (60%)

- 1-1/4 cups of whole wheat flour

- 1-1/4 cups of brown rice syrup

- 1-1/2 teaspoon vanilla extract

- 1-1/2 teaspoon cinnamon

Directions:

1. Preheat the oven to 375 °F. Cover a sheet of parchment paper for baking.

2. In a cup, whisk in the flour, oats, cinnamon, salt and baking soda. Beat the tahini and butter substitute in a mixer bowl until it is smooth. Mix in the brown rice syrup and beat until well mixed, at low speed. Beat the egg and vanilla at low speed until blended. Fold in the chocolate chips, walnuts and cranberries with a spatula when mixed.

3. On a baking sheet, drop a tablespoon of dough. Slightly flatten the dough with a fingertip. Place the dough on a cookie sheet approximately 2 inches apart. Bake for about 10-11 minutes, until it is light brown.

4. Enable to cool for 5 minutes on the baking sheet before removing.

6.4 Blueberry Bling

YIELD: 4 Servings

Ingredients

- 3 cups fresh/frozen blueberries

- 2 teaspoons butter or margarine (soft salted)

- 1 tablespoon of brown sugar

- 1 tablespoon of all-purpose flour

- ½ teaspoon cinnamon

- ½ cup oats (rolled)

Direction:

1. Preheat the oven to 375 °C.

2. Clean the blueberries, rinse them, and put them on a 9-inch pie plate.

3. Mix the butter, sugar, oatmeal, flour and cinnamon in a small bowl with a fork. Sprinkle over the blueberries with the oat mixture.

4. Bake for roughly 25 minutes. Enjoy while it is hot.

6.5 Fabulous Fig Bars

YIELD: **24** Servings

Ingredients

- 1-1/4 cups oats (old fashioned rolled)

- 1/3 cup sugar

- 1/2 cup walnuts (chopped)

- 1/4 cup of orange juice (juice from 1/2 orange)

- 1/2 cup margarine/butter (softened)

- 1-1/2 cups of all-purpose flour

- 1/2 teaspoon of baking soda

- 16-ounces dried figs (stemmed chopped)

- 2 Tablespoons of hot water

- 1 cup of packed brown sugar

- 1 large egg

Directions:

1. Preheat oven to 350 degrees. Lightly spray or oil a 9x13-inch baking pan.

2. Combine the figs, walnuts, sugar, orange juice and hot water in a mixing bowl and set aside.

3. Mix margarine and brown sugar until creamy. Add egg and mix until smooth.

4. Mix flour and baking soda. Stir into the egg mixture. Blend in oats to make a soft dough.

5. Reserve 1 cup of dough for topping. With floured fingertips, press the remaining dough into

a thin layer on the bottom of the baking pan.

6. Spread fig mixture evenly over the dough. Crumble reserved dough over the top, allowing fig mixture to show.

7. Bake 30 minutes or until golden brown. Cool completely in baking pan. Cut into 24 bars (about 2.5 x 2 inches).

6.6 Whoopie Pies

YIELD: 5 serving

Ingredients

For the cake:

- ¼ cup vegetable shortening

- ½ teaspoon of pure vanilla extract

- 1 large egg

- 1 large egg white (pasteurized)

- 1 package 18.25-ounces mixed plain chocolate cake

- 2 cups sifted confectioners' sugar

- 8 tablespoons butter (melted)

Directions:

1. Making of cakes: In the center of the oven, put a rack and preheat the oven to 350 °F. Place 2 unoiled baking sheets aside.

2. In a large mixing bowl, put the cake mix, egg and butter and beat with an electric mixer at low speed for 1 to 2 minutes until the ingredients come together in a stiff mass. Using your hands, form the dough into 1-inch balls or scoop the dough into balls. Place the dough balls on baking sheets that are 2 inches away.

3. keep baking sheets in an oven and bake up cakes for 10 to 12 minutes until they are still slightly soft. If your oven can not accommodate both baking sheets on the center rack, put one on the top

rack and one on the center rack and rotate them halfway through the baking time. Take the baking sheets from the oven and cool for 5 minutes with the cakes on them. Then move the cakes to wire racks using a metal spatula to cool fully, for 30 minutes longer.

4. Make the filling: Put the sugar, egg white, shortening, and vanilla of the confectioners in a medium-sized mixing bowl and beat at low speed with an electric mixer until it is mixed in 1 minute. Spoon about 1 teaspoon onto one cake's flat foot. To make a sandwich, cover the filling with a second cake. Repeat and serve with the remaining cakes.

6.7 Spaghetti Pie

YIELD: 3 servings

Ingredients:

- 3 large eggs

- 2 tablespoon of olive oil

- 12 oz. spaghetti (Reserve half cup of water for later)

- 1 yellow onion (chopped)

- 1 teaspoon of Chia Seeds

- 1 tablespoon dry mixed herbs (3 tbsp of fresh)

- 1 pound of ground turkey/chicken or beef)

- 1 cup of tomato paste

- 1 cup - 2% of shredded mozzarella

- 1 cup - 2% of grated Parmesan cheese

- ½ red capsicums

- ½ green capsicums

Directions:

1. Preheat the oven to 350 ºF.

2. Sauté the onions in a large skillet until tender. Add beef or ground turkey and 3⁄4 cup of tomato paste. Apply half of the pasta water and stir well with the capsicums and chia seeds.

3. Add more boiling water if needed, but consistency should be like a thick Bolognese sauce.

4. Mix the cooked pasta, parmesan cheese, eggs, 1⁄4 cup of the tomato paste and 1 cup of mozzarella in a wide dish.

5. Use the olive oil on a 9 or 10-inch pie pan.

6. Spread over the bottom of the cooking pan with the half beef mixture. To level it, apply the spaghetti mixture and press to make it flat.

7. Spread the leftover mozzarella on top, along with the remaining meat mixture.

8. Bake the pastry for 30 to 35 minutes in the oven. Please pick from the oven and leave it for about 10 minutes. Make slices with a sharp knife or pizza slicer, similar to a pie. Use a green salad while serving.

6.8 Amazing Ate-Layer Dip

YIELD: 8 servings

Ingredients

- 1 cup heated canned black beans

- 1 cup onion (diced)

- 1 ounce of Galaxy Veggie Shreds (Cheddar/another low-calorie cheese)

- 1 pouch - 4 ounces BOCA Ground Burger/another ground meat's substitute, such as Morningstar Farms version

- 10 ounces butternut squash cubes (around 2 and 1/2 cups)

- 2 cups of chopped cherry tomatoes

- 3-1/2 teaspoon of taco seasoning

- 4 cups of shredded lettuce

- 4 ounces of fat-free sour cream

- 4 ounces chopped roasted red peppers (shouldn't be packed in oil)

- lime juice, pepper & salt (Optional)

Directions:

1. Start by mixing half of the tomatoes and all the onions. Season with lime juice, salt and pepper to taste, if necessary and keep aside.

2. Then, nuke the squash with 2 tablespoons of water for 6 to 7 minutes in a sealed microwave-safe dish (until squash is soft enough to mash). Mash the squash to a pulp using a fork or a potato masher. Combine the 1-1/2 teaspoons. Season with the taco and put aside.

3. Combine the tomatoes and Boca Ground Burger and the leftover 2 tsp of taco seasoning in a skillet sprayed with nonstick spray and cook until the crumbles are defrosted, and the mixture is fully heated.

4. Place items in the following order in a broad dish: lettuce, blended tomato and onion, butternut squash, sour cream, beef blend, black beans, cheese shreds and red peppers. Serve the delicious (hot or cold).

6.9 Tomato Spinach Chicken Spaghetti

Servings: 4 servings

Ingredients

- 8-oz. fresh spinach

- 8-oz. spaghetti pasta

- 4 chopped Roma tomatoes

- 3 tablespoons of olive oil (use the high quality/oil extracted from the sun-dried tomatoes)

- 3 chopped garlic cloves

- 2 tablespoons of olive oil (drained from sun-dried tomatoes)

- 1/4 teaspoon salt

- 1/4 teaspoon salt

- 1/4 teaspoon of red pepper flakes

- 1/4 cup of sun-dried tomatoes (drained of oil)

- 1/4 cup of chopped fresh basil leaves

- 1/2 pound chopped boneless and skinless chicken (if possible, boneless and skinless thighs)

Directions:

1. On medium-low heat, add the sliced sun-dried tomatoes and 2 tablespoons of the olive oil drained from the sun-dried tomatoes to a large skillet.

2. Add a chicken (chopped) if possible; use the boneless and skinless chicken thighs, but you may also use minced chicken breast.

3. In the skillet, sprinkle red pepper flakes and salt to all the ingredients.

4. Cook for about 5 minutes on medium heat until the chicken is fully cooked and no longer pink.

5. Cover the chicken skillet with chopped fresh basil leaves, chopped tomatoes, chopped garlic and fresh spinach. Cook for around 3-5 minutes on medium heat until the spinach wilts and tomatoes secrete some of their juices. Retract from the heat.

6. Taste it, and if necessary, add more salt for taste. Close the lid to hold the heat off.

7. Following the packet instructions, cook the pasta and drain it.

8. With the vegetable and chicken, add the fried and drained pasta to the skillet.

9. Reheat at low temperature, blend properly and add more seasonings, if desired (salt and pepper). Withdraw from the sun.

You may add more high-quality olive oil at this stage while the pasta and vegetables are off-heat. It's not mandatory but is delicious indeed. Alternatively, you can apply more olive oil from the sun-dried tomato container.

6.10 Yogurt with Fresh Strawberries and Honey

YIELD: 1 serving

Ingredients:

- 4 teaspoons of honey

- 4 Tablespoons of toasted sliced almonds

- 3 cups of plain low-fat yogurt

- 1-pint strawberries (fresh)

Directions:

1. Clean and carve the strawberries into pieces and keep on side.

2. Put 3/4 cups of yogurt in each of the 4 serving plates. Divide the strawberries equally between the plates. Top each with 1 teaspoon of honey along with the topping of 1 tablespoon of toasted sliced almonds. Instantly serve now.

6.11 Pear-Cranberry Pie with Oatmeal Streusel

YIELD: 2 servings

Ingredients:

Streusel:

- 1/3 light brown sugar (packed)

- 1 tbsp unsalted butter (Chilled and small pieces)

- ¾ cup of regular oats

- ½ teaspoon of ground cinnamon

- ¼ teaspoon of ground nutmeg

Filling:

- ½ cup light brown sugar (packed)

- 2 ½ tablespoons of cornstarch

- 2 cups of fresh cranberries

- 3 cups (a half-inch) cubed (peeled / unpeeled) and 2 large pears

Remaining ingredient:

- 1 9" deep-dish pie crust (unbaked)

Directions:

1. Preheat the oven to 350 °F.

2. Combine the first 4 ingredients in a medium bowl to cook streusel; cut into butter with a pastry cutter or 2 knives till the mixture is comparable to a coarse meal.

3. Combine cranberries, 2/3 cup of brown sugar, corn starch and pear in a wide bowl to prepare the filling. So mix well to combine. Sprinkle streusel over pear mixture and spoon the pear mixture into pastry shell.

4. Cook for 1 hour at 350 degrees or it is creamy, and streusel is browned. Cool it on a wire rack for at least 1 hour.

Chapter 7 – Appetizer

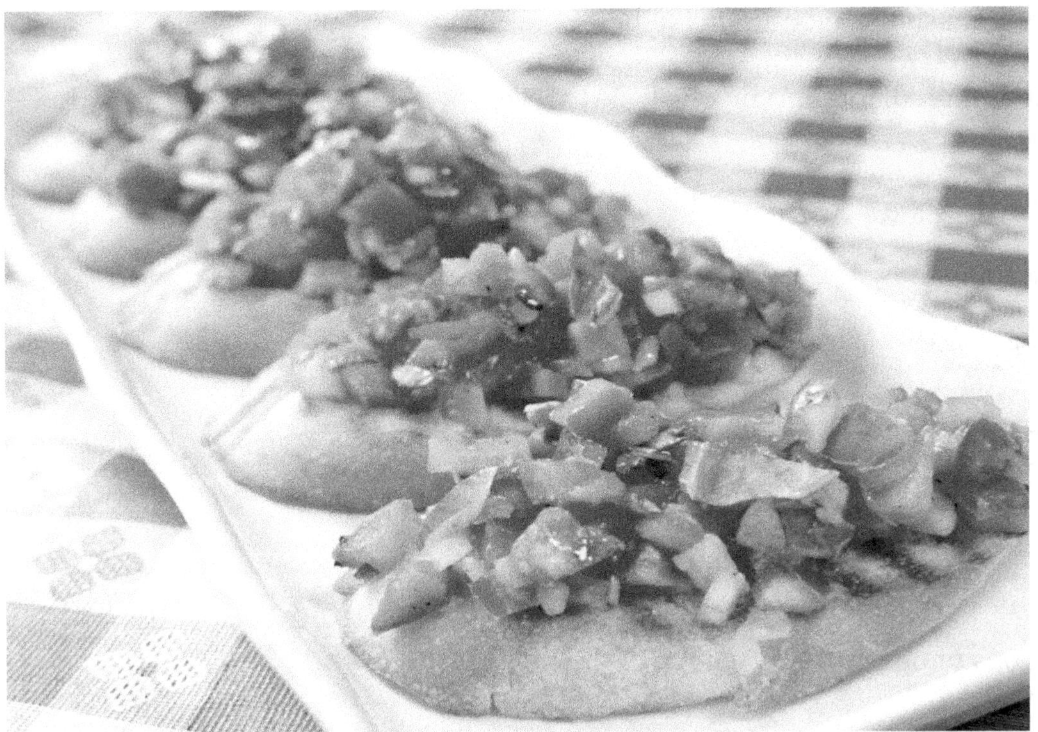

7.1 Chef Roblé Ali's Homemade Guacamole

YIELD: 4 servings

Ingredients

- pinch of cumin

- pinch of coriander

- pinch of chili powder

- 2 avocados

- 1/4 cup scallions (chopped)

- 1/2 cup tomatoes (diced)

- 1 caustic lime (cut in half)

- 1 clove garlic (chopped)

Directions:

1. Scoop and mash the avocado into a bowl.

2. Add other ingredients and mix well and serve.

7.2 Vegetable Pasta Soup

YIELD: 3 servings

Ingredients

- 12 (3/4-cup) appetizer servings

- 6 cloves minced garlic

- 4 cups of water

- 2 teaspoons of olive oil

- 2 tablespoons fresh parsley (snipped)

- 1/4 cup Parmesan cheese (shaved)

- 1 cup celery (thinly sliced)

- 1 cup onion (chopped)

- 1 32-ounce box chicken broth (reduced-sodium)

- 1 1/2 cups ditalini pasta (dried)

- 1 1/2 cups coarsen carrot (shredded)

Directions:

1. Heat the oil over medium heat in a 5 to 6 quart Dutch oven. Combine with garlic; simmer for 15 seconds. Add the onion, carrot, and celery and then roast and stir regularly for 5 -7 min until it is tender. Add the water and chicken broth and allow it to boil. Stir in uncooked pasta and boil for 7 - 8 mins or until it is tender.

2. Cover individual pieces of parsley and Parmesan cheese to eat. Allows 12 servings of (3/4-cup) appetizer.

7.3 Jamika Pessoa's Thai Peanut Salad

YIELD: 4 SERVINGS

Ingredients

- Kosher salt & black pepper (cracked)

- juice & zest (half a lime)

- 3 tablespoons of soy sauce

- 3 scallions (sliced)

- 2 tablespoon water (if needed to thin)

- 2 tablespoon rice or apple cider vinegar

- 1/4 cup lumpy peanut butter

- 1/2 teaspoon fresh/ground ginger

- 1/2 cup of cilantro leaves

- 1 tablespoon honey

- 1 cup chicken (shredded)

- 1 bag cabbage and carrot mix (shredded)

Directions

1. Put the cabbage in a serving bowl with the scallions, carrots, cilantro and chicken.

2. In a small cup, combine the remaining ingredients and whisk until combined.

3. Over the salad, pour the dressing and serve.

7.4 Bruschetta

YIELD: 2 servings

Ingredients:

- Parmesan Cheese (low fat)

- 3 tomatoes (diced)

- 2 tsp balsamic vinegar

- 2 tbsp basil (chopped)

- 2 cloves garlic (minced)

- 1/2 whole-grain bread (cut into six ½" thick diagonal pieces)

- 1 tsp olive oil

- 1 tsp black pepper

- 1 tbsp chopped parsley

Directions:

1. Toast flatbread slices until finely browned in an oven at 400 °F.

2. Mix it with all of the rest of the ingredients.

3. Blend the spoon equally over the toasted bread.

4. Topping with a little Parmesan egg.

5. Serve it while it is warm.

Conclusion

The risks of having high blood pressure or hypertension are determined by what you choose to eat.

Along with therapeutic intervention and behavioral improvements, the DASH diet seemed to be successful. In several clinical trials, the DASH diet has been well studied and found in lowering the blood pressure. DASH diet has been prescribed as the safest diet for those who wish to lose weight and reduce blood pressure. For optimal management of elevated BP, the DASH eating pattern (like other lifestyle interventions) is significant. Behavioral modifications are most commonly prescribed along with anti-hypertensive drugs, although they are regarded as a pillar of treatment.

So along with the use of the DASH diet, life changes should be in consideration. The DASH diet contains fruits, whole grains, vegetables, low-fat dairy products, fish, lean meats, and lessened sugar-sweetened desserts and some drinks that successfully decrease BP alone and in tandem with other medications. The rise in fruits and vegetables improves the diet's potassium and calcium content. DASH diet focus on lowering dietary sodium and promoting the consumption of calcium, potassium, and magnesium.

There is also evidence that the DASH diet has minimized the risk of cardiovascular heart disease, stroke, type 2 diabetes, and obesity. While vigilance should be exercised in patients with Chronic Kidney Disease (CKD), Diabetes mellitus (DM), Cardiovascular Disease (CVD), or recommended RAAS (Renin-Angiotensin-Aldosterone System) inhibitors, patient.

Therefore, for particular nutrients such as sodium, potassium, calcium, and food eaten by the population, country-specific dietary guidelines are required. In addition, for public health and clinical research, empirical studies to define the temporal correlations between the use of DASH diets and its impact on blood pressure are too essential.

Unfortunately, the diet's conformity remains poor. Studies on the long-term effectiveness of the DASH diet remain outside of clinical trials. Further research should be put on exploring the benefits of the DASH diet. Health care teams should be aware of playing their role in educating the patients about this diet's effects.

www.ingramcontent.com/pod-product-compliance
Lightning Source LLC
Chambersburg PA
CBHW081020260726
48662CB00025B/2574